Food Governs Your Destiny

Food Governs Your Destiny

The Teachings of Namboku Mizuno

Translated by Michio and Aveline Kushi
with Alex Jack

Japan Publications, Inc.
Tokyo • New York

To the Becket community
and macrobiotic friends around the world

Food Governs Your Destiny
© 1991 by Michio Kushi, Aveline Kushi, and Alex Jack

Published by Japan Publications, Inc., Tokyo & New York

Distributors:
UNITED STATES: *Kodansha International/USA, Ltd., through Farrar, Straus & Giroux, 19 Union Square West, New York 10003. CANADA: Fitzhenry & Whiteside Ltd., 195 Allstate Parkway, Markham, Ontario, L3R 4T8. BRITISH ISLES AND EUROPEAN CONTINENT: Premier Book Marketing Ltd., 1 Gower Street, London WC1E6HA. AUSTRALIA AND NEW ZEALAND: Bookwise International, 54 Crittenden Road, Findon, South Australia 5007. THE FAR EAST AND JAPAN: Japan Publications Trading Co, Ltd., 1-2-1, Sarugaku-cho, Chiyoda-ku, Tokyo 101.*

First Edition: February 1991
LCCC No. 89-63236
ISBN: 0-87040-788-0
Printed in the United States of America

Contents

Book II

Preface

Opening Words from Aveline

Growing up in Japan, my favorite study was the classics. In my autobiography, *Aveline: The Life and Dream of the Woman Behind Macrobiotics Today*, I mentioned Sontoku Ninomiya, a farmer and agricultural reformer who lived over a hundred years ago. I carried around his big book on respecting nature until the binding broke from repeated study. Recently, I discovered the writings of another great philosopher and sage, Namboku Mizuno. Mizuno is famous in Japanese history, and a long time ago I read one of his books on physiognomy. Three years ago, someone gave me Mizuno's last book, *Food Governs Your Destiny*. Michio and I were amazed at its teachings on food. He was saying exactly what we have been talking about for forty years. In his wonderful teachings, we rediscovered the meaning of our life. His dietary approach is nothing but the essence of George Ohsawa's and Michio's message. It was already stated nearly two hundred years ago.

If we really understand Mizuno's teaching, we can appreciate life, God, and spirit. There is an Oriental proverb, "Observe the old, discover the new." The meaning of this is that by studying the classics and the wisdom of the past, we can understand the pattern of present events and see the future. Like Sontoku Ninomiya, Mizuno did not depend on reading or conceptual knowledge. He discovered truth by observing nature, the book of life.

Wonderful discoveries lie ahead for you in the teachings that follow. Michio and I very much appreciate this little book. Please read it three times, as Mizuno requests, translate it into other languages, and put it into daily practice. Your life and destiny will be blessed by heaven and earth's bright shining grace.

The Life of Namboku Mizuno (1757-1825)

Mizuno's original family name was Ono. His ancestors, who traced their line scores of generations back to Heian times, included Takamuri Ono, a famous scholar, and Komachi Ono, a beautiful woman celebrated in a Noh drama. His father wrote plays in Osaka, but when he was little, Mizuno's parents died. He was brought up by an uncle who made swords and farm tools and whose family name was Mizuno. As a boy, his first name was Kuma-Taro ("Bear Boy") or sometimes Kagiya-No Kuma-Taro. Kagiya means "Locksmith," one of his uncle's skills. As a child, the boy began living up to his wild nickname. By age ten, he started drinking, fighting, and hanging out with troublemakers. He fought, argued, and disobeyed authority, giving and receiving many bruises and marks as a results of his scrapes. At age eighteen, his illegal and violent acts finally caught up with him. He was apprehended stealing money for sake — fermented rice wine — and put in jail.

Mizuno's lifelong study of physiognomy — the science of reading character and destiny in the face and other features of the human form — began in prison. In this confined setting, he began to recognize the different diagnostic signs of the other men and boys. He grew very curious about who got caught and who didn't and what kind of crimes each person had committed. Upon his release, Mizuno ran into a professional fortune-teller on the streets. The physiognomist saw clearly his troubled past and future and warned him that he would be killed in a sword fight within a year. He told him the only way to escape his fate was to become a Buddhist monk. Shaken by this prophecy, the young man presented himself at a nearby temple.

There the Zen Master knew a little physiognomy himself. Sizing up the rough youth before him, he tried to scare him away. He told him that he would accept him as a student only if he ate barley and soybeans for one year. This coarse fare was the food of the poorest peasants and sufferers of natural disaster who could not obtain rice. It would have been rejected by any usual aspirant to the monkhood. But fearful of his life, Mizuno readily agreed to the Zen Master's stipulation. Finding a job as a laborer, he ate strictly barley and soybeans as he had been told for the next twelve months.

At the end of this time, he returned to the same fortune-teller. The physiognomist was shocked at the change in Mizuno's appearance. He no longer showed signs of misfortune or early death. "The trouble with the sword has all disappeared," he told the grateful youth. "You have accumulated much wonderful merit." After hearing Mizuno's story, the fortune-teller attributed the change in his appearance to his austerities, not the meager food itself.

This was the turning point in Mizuno's life. From this time on, he grew confident that he would live and make something of his life. Rather than returning to the Zen monastery, however, he started traveling the length and breadth of Japan, and at about age twenty-one embarked on a period of self-study. Determined to become a physiognomist, he sought out anyone who could teach him this art, including Shinto priests, Buddhist monks, Confucian scholars, and *sennin*, the legendary free men who lived in the mountains and were said to have discovered the secrets of immortality. Some of these adventures, including the story of how he came to be named Namboku, are told in Book III of the present volume.

In addition to his wilderness sojourns, Mizuno lived and worked for periods in Osaka and other large cities. In order to perfect the art of physiognomy, he served as an apprentice to a hairdresser for three years, studying heads, faces, and hands. Next, he worked as an attendant at a public bath house for three years, scrubbing people's bodies. Finally, he studied bone structure and anatomy working at a mortuary for three years, handling corpses and cremating remains.

After nine years of careful observation, he began to practice physiognomy and fortune-telling. The accuracy of his predictions attracted attention, and his reputation spread. But Mizuno was still dissatisfied. Although he had mastered the traditional methods of visual diagnosis, he recognized that something was lacking. Eventually, he made a pilgrimage to the Ise Shrine. The Ise Shrine is the great national shrine of Japan, where millions of people, including the Imperial family, traditionally worship. Located in a beautiful forest with tall, majestic cedar trees, the graceful inner temple of Ise is dedicated to the Goddess of Grain and Food. After three weeks of training by the Ksuzu River, fasting and bathing in cold water each day, Mizuno attained satori. He discovered that people's destiny is governed by their daily food. The wonderful order in human lives and cultures is not fixed but ever-changing. It is dependent principally on the quality and quantity of

9

food consumed.

Settling in Atsuta, near Nagoya, Mizuno built a house and welcomed his clients with cheap tea and meager food so that he could study their reaction. People from all backgrounds and ways of life came to his door — aristocratics and geisha, samurai and priests, wealthy landowners and gangsters, intellectuals and sumo wrestlers, the mentally gifted and the mentally ill. In time, Mizuno became the most famous physiognomist of his time and wrote a dozen books on diagnosis and fortune-telling.

Mizuno himself was very frugal in his daily way of eating. As he explains in this book, he ate about one and a half cups of barley or wheat each day, along with a cup of sake, and side dishes of miso soup and a small plate of vegetables. He didn't eat rice which was then the most luxurious grain. Nor did he eat mochi — pounded sweet rice traditionally served on New Year's and other special occasions. By his own account, Mizuno's physiognomy was very poor. In appearance, he was very yang — short, compacted, and ugly. His mouth was small. His eyes were piercing and deeply sunk. His forehead was small, and his eyebrows very thin and shallow. He had a flat nose, high cheeks, small stubby teeth, and small feet.

Despite these unenviable features, Mizuno extended his own lifespan by many decades, while many around him with more beautiful countenances led short, unhappy lives. Of his family life, little is known. He is said to have married a wife who was beautiful but proud, a combination that may account for his general low regard for women. He accumulated much wealth over the years and ended up with a large house and seven storerooms to keep his treasures. His son, Yoshikuni, was reportedly spoiled by the mother and used up all his possessions. Mizuno passed away on November 11, 1825. He was sixty-eight. He received an honorary title, Dai-Nippon, from the Emperor Kokaku.

Mizuno's Times

Mizuno lived during the Tokugawa Era, an epoch of relative peace and prosperity spanning nearly three centuries between the end of the feudal wars and Japan's entrance into the modern world. During this period of tranquility and isolation, Japan remained a predominantly agricultural country with a spiritual orientation to life and respect for traditional values. But by the time Mizuno was born, change had already set in, and the time-honored Japanese way of life, associated with Shinto ceremony, Buddhist piety, Confucian order, and the samurai code, was being challenged by urbanization and the emergence of new lifestyles and values. The period from 1680 to 1740, the generation of Mizuno's parents and grandparents, was known as *Genroku* or Cafe Society. It was the Golden Age of luxurious kimono shops, narrow lanes decorated with paper lanterns, crowded theaters featuring revolving stages, dainty tea houses, and ostentatious pleasure gardens. It is the period of the *Ukiyo-e,* or Floating World, celebrated in the woodcuts of Hiroshige and Hokusai. Drifting through this colorful current of life were wives and courtesans in glossy coiffures, actors and rakes decked out in gaudy fabrics, newly rich merchants and vain scions of wealthy houses, worldly monks and priests, and envious farmers and peasants seeking to exchange the natural rhythms of the country for the artificial stimulants of urban life.

From time immemorial, the Japanese had recognized the impermanence of all things and come to appreciate the fleeting beauty of life. During the *Genroku*, the country's traditional acceptance of life's brevity and viscissitudes gave way to indulgence and pleasure-seeking. The best-selling books of the day were *The Man Who Spent His Life in Love, Twenty Examples of Unfilial Conduct,* and *Characters of Worldly Young Men.* In Kyoto, the capital, Osaka, the mercantile center, Edo, the residence of the shogunate (the real seat of power), and other big cities, the aristocracy and rising middle class increasingly enjoyed rich gourmet foods, gold-lacquered serving dishes, and an unreflective way of eating that emphasized sensory taste and elaborate presentation. There is the story told of Kinokuniya Bunzaemon, a rich merchant, who had the staircase to his tea-house widened so that an enormous pastry could be delivered to his upstairs chambers. In the rapidly multiplying cafes, banquet halls, taverns, and pleasure houses, men and women, young and the old, refined and rustic, celebrated the ephemerality of life listening to the lute, gambling with dice and cards, and feasting on rich octopus meat and fish paste, polished rice and aromatic spices, and endless bowls of sake.

Like a firecracker, this period of impressionism briefly lit up the

Japanese cultural sky. By Mizuno's time, economic pressures, natural cycles of flood and drought, the growing political ascendancy of Edo (modern-day Tokyo), and the revolt of the intelligentsia to the country's self-imposed isolation from the rest of the world had caused the glitter to fade. Once again, the Japanese, like most people, were preoccupied with the practical concerns of daily life. Still the trends and precedents of the *Genroku* made deep inroads in the Japanese character. Mizuno's frequent references to people with "floating minds" show the extent of this rootless, transitory, modern way of thinking.

Mizuno's Teaching

Mizuno is both a product of this transient world — as his early life attests — and the world of ceaseless order and permanency. He is representative of the prophet who comes out every few generations to warn society that it is headed toward self-destruction He is the sage who guides people back to health, happiness, and peace through an understanding of the universal laws of change and balance. In Japan, we also find this figure in Ekiken Kaibara, the Confucian educator, who lived about a century before Mizuno. Kaibara's book, *Yojokun*, translated into English as *Japanese Secrets of Good Health* (Tokyo: Tokuma Shoten, 1974), had a far-reaching influence on instilling moral values and principles of moderation within Tokugawa society.   In Sontoku Ninomiya, the Peasant Saint who lived about a generation after Mizuno and who taught farmers to pool their resources for mutual aid, we find another representative of this archetype. In our own day, we might include George Ohsawa, the founder of modern macrobiotics, and Masanobu Fukuoka, the natural farmer and author of *The One-Straw Revolution*, in this category.

Like Kaibara before him and Ninomiya, Ohsawa, and Fukuoka after him, Mizuno came to a deep understanding of yin and yang — the principles of balance and harmony — and applied them to the problems and concerns at hand. In his case, the field was physiognomy, the traditional art of visual diagnosis. Over the course of history, especially in China where schools of face-reading and fortune-telling had existed for centuries, physiognomy had become an exact science with fixed rules and procedures. The same happened in respect to astrology, numerology, geomancy, and other sacred arts, in addition, of course, to religion and philosophy as a whole. Shinto, Confucianism, and Buddhism had lost much of their original freshness and vitality and were practiced in name only or in very formal or stylized ways.

At an early age, Mizuno learned that there were exceptions to the physiognomic art. One's fate was not set in stone. Like Dostoevski, who was pardoned just before facing a firing squad for youthful insurrectionary activities, or like Dr. Tony Sattilaro, who was recalled by life after being diagnosed with terminal cancer throughout his body, Mizuno came to revolutionize his chosen field of study in gratitude for the gift of life and opportunity to master his own destiny. This is his deepest teaching — even beyond the way of eating that is his major concern. Life is not set or predetermined. Our future is not engraved in the stars or our countenances. Character and destiny are not predetermined and unalterable. Of course, a past pattern is there, tendencies are established, probabilities exist. But the lines of our face and hands, the blood that courses through our vessels and organs, the *ki* or natural electromagnetic energy that pulsates through our meridians and chakras, can all be changed. Life is free, life is flowing, life is ever new and renewing itself.

Like Kaibara, Ninomiya, Ohsawa, and Fukuoka, Mizuno teaches that the most effective way to realize this freedom and happiness is through dietary practice — the proper way of growing, selecting, and preparing our daily foods. In Mizuno's day, food quality was generally good. Rice and other grains, for the most part, were whole and unrefined. Beans and bean products (such as tofu and miso), vegetables, seaweed, fruits, and other foods were not grown with chemicals or treated with artificial additives. The principal animal products consumed were fish and seafood. It was not until the Meiji Era, several generations later after the country was opened by gunboat diplomacy, that the Japanese government began to encourage people to eat meat, dairy food, and eggs in order to compete aggressively with the West. Also, because of Japan's isolation, sugar, spices, and other tropical foods from Taiwan and Southeast Asia that made their entrance into the country by the late nineteenth century, were absent from the Tokugawa dining table.

In this social milieu, where macrobiotic food was widely eaten, Mizuno was concerned less with the quality of food consumed than with the way in which it is eaten. In particular, he warned against overeating and disorderly eating — eating at irregular times and in irregular ways. Beyond the important health benefits of eating small amounts of food in an orderly manner, Mizuno concentrates on the mental, emotional, and spiritual effects of our daily way of eating that we often overlook. His philosophy is at once simple and profound. It is hard to regard money the same after studying his observations on the relation between food and income. Or take the matter of saving food. Most of us have been conditioned to see food in exclusively material terms, sort of "a grain saved is a grain earned." Mizuno teaches us that the macrobiotic motto, "one grain, ten thousand grains," applies to the invisible world. Every grain we save actually results in saving ten thousand grains. By reducing our daily food, if only by one mouthful a meal, we are saving thousands and thousands of grains and reaping countless blessings.

Mizuno's Significance for Our Era

As a forefather of modern macrobiotics, we find many familiar terms and concepts in Mizuno's pages. In addition to yin and yang, his basic vocabulary includes heaven's and earth's force, *ki* energy, condition and constitution, the tao (Japanese *do*), karma, and reincarnation. In his language and speech, he is both contemporary and timeless. The image we get is of a very salty sage holding court to ailing merchants and indolent students, upwardly mobile samurai and hapless suitors — a combination of George Ohsawa and Ann Landers. It is easy to imagine sitting down across from Mizuno and being transfixed by his penetrating gaze as he gauges our reaction to the meager tea and refreshment he has set before us. It is not hard to discern the warm heart behind his blunt exterior. If he has a major flaw, it is his view of woman. Possibly because of his own experience, as well as the lingering effects of the samurai heritage, his views on woman are colored by a basic mistrust. Rather than appreciating the wonderful complemental-antagonism of woman's and man's natures, he accepts man's more stable, rational energy as the yardstick for evaluating all human development. Woman's more spontaneous, intutitive energy is a necessary balance in the dance of the sexes. It is not surprising that Mizuno's own household lacked family unity as a consequence of this limited view. In this respect, macrobiotics continues to evolve and grow with each era and generation.

Another omission in the pages that follow is any reference to the West. But this is not surprising considering the near total isolation of the time. Still, to put Mizuno and his age in perspective, it is useful to recall that in 1807, the year the book was written, on the other side of the world, in the newly formed United States of America, Thomas Jefferson was president. Interestingly, Jefferson who introduced brown rice into Virginia (smuggling it in from Italy), Franklin, and other more macrobiotically-oriented statesmen were the last generation of culture-bearers on the North American continent to recognize the primacy of agriculture and the importance of a grain-centered diet on individual health and national destiny. Mizuno's horizon extends only as far as India and China. But his view of the unity of all religions is truly planetary in scope. The entire world, as he states, is "God's country."

The glittering society of the *Genroku* has long disappeared, but much of the modern world, led increasing by Japan, is embracing a global culture based on instant gratification and excess. Like physiognomy in its day, medicine and science in our own, are largely fixed disciplines, lacking in *ki* or natural vitality. As Mizuno rediscovered the truth of physiognomy, so it is up to those of us today who are macrobiotic educators and teachers to renew medicine and science and make them once again living, breathing arts in the service of life. Whatever our interest or abilities, Mizuno's wonderful book will inspire us to study nature and society and to discover the invincible laws of change. The virtues he embraces — hard work, perseverance, patience, modesty, and concealing our merits — are not fashionable. But what is currently in season will soon pass, as the Spiral of History reaches its climax, and the planet enters a new cycle of comprehensive growth and development. Mizuno's spirit can help guide us toward that radiant new era of universal health, happiness, and peace which is humanity's ultimate destiny.

The Translation

In Japanese, the name of the book is *So Ho Gokui Syu Shin Roku*. *So Ho* means "diagnose." *Gokui* means "secret of." *Syu Shin* is "way of life," and *Roku* is "text" or "book." The literal translation is "The Book of the Secret of Diagnosing Way of Life." The subtitle is translated as "Food Destiny Left/Right Changes." Left/right refers to yin/yang — the universal forces of expansion and contraction that make up all things. We have translated this as "Food Governs Your Destiny."

The present volume is based on two versions of the Japanese original, one an older unabridged edition; the other a modern, abridged one. Keiji Yamaguchi, a journalist and macrobiotic teacher based in Philadelphia, assisted in the translation for which we are very grateful. The end result, it is hoped, conveys the spirit of the original without sacrificing too much of the author's pithy style and rhythm.

Footnotes have been added and grouped at the back to provide information on some special terms, people, and places mentioned in the text. A reading list for further study is also included in addition to information on seminars and classes at the Kushi Institute of the Berkshires that offer further study of Mizuno's teachings.

We are grateful to our families, associates, and students for their support, suggestions, and encouragement during the course of this project. We are especially thankful to Mr. Iwao Yoshizaki and Mr. Yoshiro Fujiwara, president and vice-president of Japan Publications, for their unswerving devotion to macrobiotic publishing and to Gale Jack, Alex's wife, for proof-reading.

As Aveline tells her students, Mizuno's book represents "the essence of the essence of macrobiotics." It belongs in every home, school, and office. When the new One Peaceful World Inn is completed in Becket, copies will be put in every room like Gideon Bibles. We hope that you read *Food Governs Human Destiny* and act upon its teachings to help realize our common dream of one healthy, peaceful world.

Michio and Aveline Kushi
Alex Jack
One Peaceful World Village
Becket, Massachusetts
February, 1990

Food Governs Your Destiny

The Teachings of Namboku Mizuno

Translated by Michio
& Aveline Kushi
with Alex Jack

Introduction

The origin of human life is food. Though we take many wonderful medicines, we cannot survive without eating. Humanity's true, wonderful medicine is food. For many years, I have devoted myself to diagnosing people and telling their fortune. But I didn't know the value of food. Sometimes I saw people who were born with poor physiognomic features indicating suffering and a short life, but still they were rich, happy, and long-lived. Similarly, I saw others with very good diagnostic features indicating wealth, nobility, and longevity, but in reality they were very poor, suffering, and lived only a short life.

I talked about fortune and misfortune, but from physiognomy I couldn't read people's destinies clearly and predict the future. But recently, I have gradually begun to understand the real origin and development of fortune and misfortune. I found that whether we eat food greedily in great quantity or in small volume with humility and respect is the key to eating. When I see people, the first thing I now ask them is how much they eat — a large or small amount. From their answer, I can diagnose their destiny in life accurately. Even in ten thousand cases, I won't make a mistake.

For a few years, I have been teaching people to be modest and humble in their food and drink and am using this method to give them advice. This is the deep essence of my way of physiognomy. Even if they face great difficulty in the year ahead, if they pay attention to their way of eating they can escape their problems. Besides avoiding future problems or tragedy, some people experience unexpected good fortune at the time of their year of difficulty as a result of changing their way of eating. Such people are many. Or someone whose physical structure indicates a lifetime of poverty and misery will become happy and rich by using this method. They get a suitable reward, and people notice their good fortune. Such people are many. In many cases, people who have been weak, chronically sick, and facing a short life become healthy in body and mind. If they are moderate in their food, they are now still alive and enjoying life. There are many such people among the rich and noble and among the poor and low grade. I can't even begin to count such examples I have seen. Longevity and short life, suffering and happiness — all aspects of human life depend on modesty in food and drink. That is why I sincerely wish you will read this book and observe a modest, humble way of eating.

I myself have not eaten rice my whole life or even eaten things made with rice such as mochi. My daily food is barley, and I eat altogether about 1 1/2 cups a day. I enjoy sake very much, but I limit myself to only one cup a day. I don't cut down on food just for myself, but for society. I wish to inspire some sincere person, even only for one day, to please be moderate in their food and drink.

I was born into poverty and a low grade of society. My personality wasn't very sociable. But because of my humble way of eating, I gradually entered a group of physiognomists. I have founded my own school of diagnosis, and now from among my eight books I have gathered four chapters on food for this present volume. But I'm foolish and ignorant. Some misuse of words may arise in this book, and my expression may be awkward or funny. But please do not be put off by my strange explanations. I can say again and again, please read this book three times. After that you can form your own ideas. Please don't be careless, laugh, or throw this book away.

There are Confucian scholars who like to write beautiful words and play around with ideas and concepts. These people don't have a real impact on society. Such persons may read my book and foolishly dismiss it. Great people understand and teach ordinary people. That way such persons criticize this book and are enemies of the Tao. They don't harmonize with heaven's order and are never able to succeed in society. They think they are great, but ordinary people don't respect them, and society doesn't follow them. You can observe such people. Heaven naturally punishes them. Please, yourself, be modest and humble.

Namboku Mizuno

Book I

The quantity of food eaten — big or small — governs health, wealth, longevity, and our future destiny.

#1 Food Determines One's Destiny

A. What I'm writing now applies only for those who are not engaged in very much physical labor. Those who do vigorous physical work have their own appropriate amount of food to eat according to their work and the size and strength of their body. The principle does not apply to young people either, especially those who are not the head of the household. But even if they are young and master of the family, their destiny is determined by the amount of food they eat.

An old proverb says, "Everyone is born with heaven's blessing just as every plant has its roots in the ground." Being born into a rich or poor family doesn't really matter, because the exact quantity of food we need for this life has been determined by heaven. This explains the proverb, "If someone overeats the food provided by heaven, his conduct is against heaven's order." Those who do not know their place in society and eat greedily are breaking heaven's law. Every living thing has its own fixed amount of food provided by heaven. Where there is life, sufficient food always follows. We look at it the other way around. But actually food precedes us. Wherever there is life, there is food, and wherever there is food, there is life. In short, food is the origin of life. Food is the essence of life, and everything we do is governed by how we eat. We should always hold food in the deepest respect. We have to be modest in our way of eating. Food is really of the greatest importance.

B. The Amount of Food and Longevity and Wealth

If someone with poor physiognomy eats less than the amount of food given to him by heaven, he will enjoy a life of good fortune. He can attain prosperity and longevity. In old age, he will be happy. If someone with good physiognomic features eats more than the fixed amount of food given by heaven, he will find many difficulties in life. His hands tend to become numb, troubles arise in the end of the nervous system, and tiredness and stress will disturb his whole life. Old age is especially miserable.

#2 A Person of Meager Food, Even with Poor Physiognomy, Can Attain a Happy Life

A. If your food is in the right amount, your destiny will be just as your physiognomy shows.

B. People who overeat, even with good physiognomic features, will have rather unsteady lives. Poor people like this will become poorer. Even wealthy people who overeat will destroy their house and family. People with poor features will be buried without a coffin.

C. One who enjoys rich food beyond his limit, even with good physiognomy, will attract big misfortune. Unless he is careful, he will destroy his house. He cannot progress and prosper all through his life. A poor man who likes rich food will have to work hard to make ends meet and experience many difficulties until the end of his life.

One who enjoys early food harvested at the beginning of the season, even with good physiognomy, will lose his wealth and destroy his house. One with poor physiognomy will use up his grace and end up wandering far from home.

E. One who eats less than his limit, even with poor physiognomy, will find wealth, longevity, and enjoy good fortune in old age.[1]

#3 Overeating Even Occasionally Brings Bad Fortune Even to a Person Who Eats Simply

A. A person who eats a small amount of simple food, even with the worst physiognomy, can attain wealth and longevity as well as accumulate enough wealth for his descendants and become famous even after his death. Nevertheless, if he sometimes overeats even simple food, he will find great misfortune. Country people are an exception to this rule.

B. One who strictly controls his food, even with bad physiognomy, will progress and surely attain wealth. His house and family will continue to prosper. Also later in life he will enjoy good fortune and happiness.

C. One who strictly controls his food by taking a small amount, even with bad physiognomy, will gradually accumulate wealth and enjoy a long life. He will obtain heaven's grace, and everything he imagines will be realized later in life. The course of his life will be steady. Such a person may look very weak, but inside he is very strong. Also he usually won't get sick.

#4 Irregular Eating Attracts Bad Luck Even to a Person with Good Physiognomy

A. One who eats at irregular meal times, even with good physiognomy, will have bad fortune. Somehow he cannot accomplish things in life and can never set his mind at rest. One who eats this way, with poor physiognomic features, tends to experience a breakdown after completing 80 to 90 percent of his goal. These people accomplish little and, as a result, get tired physically and mentally and injure their mind and life.

B. If one is both a big eater and an irregular eater, it is useless to discuss his fate. Unless he becomes modest, he will lose everything and become sick. Further, if his physiognomy is bad to begin with, he won't have a suitable place to die.

#5 Eating a Regular Quantity of Food Ensures Health of Mind and Body

A. A person whose quantity of food is regular but from time to time eats a little bit irregularly will find that his income becomes unstabilized. A steady amount of food makes for a steady income. Only strict control of the amount of food consumed and eating at regular times brings good fortune. A person who eats aggressively and disorderly cannot have a steady and quiet mind and therefore can't manage anything. Such a person, even with good physiognomy, cannot attain anything in life at all and wanders around unless he changes his eating pattern.

A person who eats regularly can manage himself well and maintain a steady mind which will enable him to manage most things well. A head of a wealthy house should know that his inherited wealth will not last if he eats a lot and eats chaotically. He cannot sustain this way of life very long without eating up his wealth and health. We can confidently make this prediction. Moreover, if the servants of such a person overeat following the example of their master, the house will decline even sooner. On the outside, a person may look nice and appear to be managing himself well and be wealthy, but inside his life is not even and calm and his income will be unsteady.

Income corresponds to diet. Unless food is strictly controlled and stabilized, the income cannot be stabilized. Therefore such a person cannot manage his daily life well, and his future is dark.

B. A person who eats simply and observes the limit of food given to him by heaven will have no great misfortunes in life. Women eat less than men and suffer fewer big troubles as a result. Sometimes a person who is very strong and courageous is a big eater. Those people we call Big Food Guys. The tendency is for people around them to be cautious. They are not really virtuous. In contrast, someone who eats very strictly, limiting his quantity of food for daily life, enjoys people's true respect. People see his true heart and admire him. He is virtuous and easy to trust.

C. If the woman overeats, we say she "suppresses her husband."[2] She should know overeating may destroy her marriage. Such a woman is eating man's style. Her *ki* energy becomes too strong and she ends up sitting on top of her husband. Then if the man is also strong, she cannot get on top of him, and they divorce.

A woman who eats simply but controls her husband is a bad wife. She goes from lover to lover and makes her husband suffer.

D. If a person who eats regularly starts to eat irregularly, misfortune or an accident may occur. He should correct his eating pattern quickly to restore order.

When the household is in disorder, people tend to eat chaotically and misfortune arises. Of course, family troubles are also the result of past difficulties in eating. In case the way of eating becomes irregular without any household troubles around, this is the sign of impending bad fortune.

When a person who is going to inherit family wealth starts indulging in rich food every day without any humility, that is a sure sign of the decline of the house or that he will retire very soon.

E. A person who looks very orderly and refined but eats in a disorderly way has a weak mind and spirit. He is only decorating the outside. A person who controls his food has a strong mind. As a result of his way of eating, his outlook becomes even more orderly. A person with good looks outside but a weak mind inside is very superficial.

F. A person who has observed a disciplined way of eating from an early age won't have any sicknesses or difficulties. He will progress in society and encounter strong good fortune. Such a person, even with bad physiognomy, will be all right. The older he grows, the happier he will become.

G. A person who eats aggressively and disorderly, even with good physiognomy, will undoubtedly face misfortune. A noble person is right and doesn't eat a lot. A low or small person does not know his limit and eats aggressively. It's been said that a big or great person eats and then understands the order of heaven, while a small person overeats, forgets himself, and engages in misconduct. Therefore, one who eats little makes himself naturally noble.

H. When a person who has been eating only a small amount of food feels sick and can't eat, he will soon die, even if his pulse and face color are normal. Such a person has eaten up all the food given by heaven and, as in this case, dies without any suffering or sickness.

I. If an upper class person likes meager food and eats a lot of this, his mind will change to that of a peasant. He will have a short life. Everyone has an amount of food to eat that matches with their rank. Lower class people usually should eat a simple diet of grains and one side dish.

J. A noble man should not eat meager food. Nevertheless, if he has a small amount of meager food out of humility, his house will prosper with the grace extended from nature. Such a master of a house will make a great name for himself, which his descendants can be proud of, enjoy a long, healthy life, and remain free from sickness.

K. A sick person younger than fifty, even with physiognomic signs of approaching death, may overcome his fate if he limits his food to a small amount.[3] He can live on. His difficulties comes not from sickness, but from astrological or directional influences.[4]

Food is the origin of life. Someone who eats a small amount won't become sick. Therefore, his suffering must come because of a bad direction. Medicine is no use in such a case. A person who eats such a small amount uses up less grain. This way of eating will accumulate grace from heaven and earth. Such a person will not die because of traveling in a bad direction. I have witnessed such cases several times.

L. Generally when a person over fifty-seven or fifty-eight develops serious illness, even with physiognomic signs of longevity and a healthy face color, he may die if he has been eating aggressively and disorderly. There are many people who die not because their supposed life span ends but because they have eaten up the food allotted to them by heaven at birth. Therefore it's not easy to determine one's life span from looking only at his physiognomy. There is no mistake if you judge from finding out what he eats. Therefore, when you see a sick person, ask him what his diet is to determine his health and destiny.

#6 Eating Gourmet Food for a Long Time Makes Sickness in the Digestive System

A. A person with no diagnostic signs of ill health who has been indulging in rich food every day from an early age will develop sickness in the *hara*, which makes him unable to eat.[5] Such a person with little virtue in the beginning will destroy his house and therefore won't be able to eat rich food any longer. Even if he escapes sickness, he will have bad fortune in old age. Whether his physiognomy is good or bad, such is the inevitable result of eating rich food. If you are a lower class person and eat rich food for three years, you will lose your happiness in old age and die.

B. You should know that even with good physiognomy, someone will not be able to accomplish anything in life if he indulges in rich food from an early age. Please do not be mislead by only good physiognomy. Waning follows waxing. This is the order of heaven and earth.

A person who eats aggressively and disorderly without any humbleness will not progress nor prosper in life. He will find nowhere to lie down to die. People who are working very hard physically are an exception to this rule.

But a person with good physiognomy and wealth may find a place to lie down and die, but people will not like him and he will suffer very much. He will also be sick for a long time. A poor person with bad physiognomy will find no one to help or take care of him on his death bed. He cannot even have a last drink of water at his death.

C. A person between middle age and early old age who has not yet stabilized his food pattern will experience misfortune from time to time, trouble, or an accident, and then fall back. He will always be tired both physically and mentally for the rest of his life.

D. Such a person, even with good physiognomy, will find that his house declines, and he will never be able to prosper. *Ki* energy depends on food. Without managing your eating pattern well, you cannot control the *ki* within yourself. If your daily eating is disorderly, then nothing can be managed, and misfortune or an accident arises. Naturally you cannot prosper. Therefore controlling one's food is the essence of human life. When your food is under control, your *ki* is settled, peaceful, and quiet, and you are able to keep your mind under control. No accident will happen to someone with such a steady and harmonious mind. Naturally, it's then easy to manage the household.

E. A person whose physiognomy indicates misfortune in old age can still enjoy a happy life if he is humble in his eating from an early age. Then he can avoid tragedy in his later years. One can avoid any misfortune by being modest and humble and extending his grace to old age.

Even an old man with physiognomic signs of dying of starvation could avoid his fate by eating very humbly for three years and using up less of the food given to him at birth by heaven. I know some examples. An old person with a bad physiognomy should be modest in order to enjoy his later days.

#7 Even If You Are Destined to Be Childless, You Can Have One with Modest Eating

A. If your physiognomy shows that you won't have children, by eating strictly and not taking large quantities of food you can find a very able child to adopt.[6] If one eats simply and orderly from a young age, he can extend his virtue to heaven and earth beyond what he has been given at birth. This extended virtue will return to him in old age as an heir. Therefore, even if lonely now, he will find a child. Even after death, there will be someone to serve food to your spirit.[7] Even a wealthy man without a child looks poor and finds difficulties in old age. Children are a treasure who can nourish you in years to come.

B. Even with good physiognomy now, if a person indulges in

food and drink, he will not be able to sustain his wealth. When a prosperous person floods himself with food, his grace begins to wane. Even with wealth, one should be as modest as a poor man. Then he can accomplish things very well. Nevertheless, ebbing and flowing repeat in everything. Therefore, "wealth" is also "decline."[8] At the peak of waning, waxing begins. That's why they say the extravagant will not last long.[9]

C. Even a person with the best physiognomic signs of longevity will not live long if he eats a lot and eats irregularly. Food nourishes life. Unstable eating nourishes only unstable life. That is the reason why he cannot attain longevity. A person with proper food can nourish his life properly and live long. By being modest in eating one can hold longevity. Unless you are modest, you cannot live long even with good diagnostic signs of longevity.

D. Even with physiognomic signs of poverty and a short life, a man can avoid this fate if he is modest and eats less than the amount of food given to him by heaven. A person who is modest in food is also modest in not wasting anything. Therefore, his food and wealth accumulates and becomes full in heaven and earth, and he can naturally extend his life and wealth. Therefore, even with physiognomic signs of poverty and a short life you can attain happiness and a long life by being frugal.

E. We should say that a person, even with physiognomic signs of great success and prosperity, cannot prosper by being lazy, enjoying meat and sake, and not working hard at whatever they do. Such people tend to float through life and exhaust the nourishment given to them by heaven.

Even without any physiognomic signs of success, if you really want to progress in life, then you can easily achieve this by concentrating on your work, strictly controlling your eating, and avoiding rich food until your goal is attained.

But if you enjoy this kind of food and have a floating mind, you will never to able to reach your goal. Food is the origin of success. If your way of eating is disorderly, you are ruining the origin and will not succeed in the end. Please think of the importance of food. Be careful.

Gold and silver certainly have great virtue. But nothing has greater virtue than the five grains.[10] The wealth of lords is all measured not by their amount of gold or silver but by the amount of rice they possess.[11] The Emperor prays for an abundant harvest of the five grains. We should approach food with great reverence. There are times when the market cost of things goes up sharply. But inflation cannot result in chaos in the country. Only poor and improper management of the five grains can bring disturbance to people and to society.

#8 A Small Eater Doesn't Have Long Sicknesses Nor Suffering at Death

A. A big eater cannot eat from the beginning of his illness. A small eater seldom gets sick. Even when he becomes ill, he does not lose his appetite for food. A big eater has eaten up the food which was given to him at birth. Therefore, his life remains but there is no more food. He has to suffer a long time and dies without being able to eat. His death is just like hunger and will be a very painful one in contrast. Because a small eater has been extending his food and virtue to heaven and earth, he can extend his life beyond his destined life span. His food supply still remains. That's why life continues. Such is the order of nature. If our food supply ends, life automatically ceases. But if food is still there, life automatically follows. Therefore, a small eater will have no pain at death, nor long sicknesses. But a small eater will become sick if he eats irregularly. A big eater cannot eat when sickness comes because his stomach is always full. A small eater, because his stomach is not full, can eat when sick and naturally does not develop any serious illness.

B. Those who earn a steady income always have steady meals three times a day.

C. Those whose income is not stable are those who cannot regulate their food well.

D. Those who cannot earn a steady salary are lower class people, people who stay in hostels, and laborers. They cannot realize a steady income because of irregular and disorderly eating. Therefore, one who wants to have a stable income must regulate his food at first. If he wants a high salary, then he must eat a small volume and modestly. Such a person, even with physiognomic signs of poverty, can regulate his income after eating modestly for three years. I tried this method in some people with success. Food is the beginning of income. Unsteady food makes unsteady income. By strictly regulating one's food, he can regulate his income. Therefore, there are no good or bad physiognomic signs. Controlling one's eating and drinking alone can make good physiognomy. Unless one's food is regulated, I must say his physiognomy is bad. It's best to eat only to eighty percent capacity. But this rule doesn't apply to samurai.[12]

Food for Samurai

E. Many samurai are strong and big eaters. Generally, this is not bad. During peaceful times, society is governed by Shintoism, Confucianism, and Buddhism, and they study those teachings. But when society falls into chaos, war begins. It is the demon's way to conquer by fighting and life turns evil. It is the samurai's job to restore order in society. When chaos arrives, samurai have to fight for society and can't always eat food. That's why they are bigger, in order to store up food in their body and organs. Even during ordinary times, they have to eat more quantity than usual. They eat this way not to satisfy their personal wishes but for society and the country. In an emergency, such big and strong eating is permissible. Real, true samurai are strict in their way of eating and eat big quantities only when necessary. Such a warrior sets a good example. His personality is also big and great.

F. A high ranking samurai who consumes great quantities and is not orderly in his way of eating will spoil his fighting spirit, become distracted, and encounter a strange destiny and difficulties. He also has to retire early. Unless he becomes humble, he will lose his position and income. This does not apply to samurai who are foolish but eat strongly. For a samurai to realize health and prosperity, he must eat strictly and orderly at first and once or twice a month take a lot of simple food to expand his stomach. This is a samurai's humbleness. With such humbleness, he can manage well. Thinking of the difficult wartimes which his lord and ancestors had to go through, a samurai must be careful not to take it easy in peacetime. If a samurai constantly reflects on this, his conduct follows heaven's order, and he can progress.

G. Even a samurai born into a family of high rank cannot progress if he does not take care of food, overeats, and follows a disorderly way of eating.[13] Nevertheless, being humble in his eating, he can progress to a commanding position. Needless to say, a samurai should be good and strong and master the tao of swordsmanship. But being more proficient in swordplay doesn't make him any more successful. A samurai receives his food three times a day every day from his lord as his salary.[14] Therefore, a samurai who is disorderly and overeats is destroying his salary which is given by his lord. He is not respecting the lord. This behavior is against the tao of a samurai. The samuari's tao is to respect the food given to him by his lord and to eat properly with respect for the virtue of the lord. Such a samurai will certainly progress to high rank. Once again, good physiognomy is not judged by structure and appearance but by way of eating. That is the essence.

#9 It Is Permissable for a Hard Laborer to Be a Big Eater

A. It is permissible for someone who is very physically active and hard-working to eat a large amount of food. It looks like he is working only for himself, but he is also working for society. Unless he eats a lot, he cannot fulfill his duty. Be aware of this. He is like a Bodhisattva and feeding his wife and children.[15] He must, though, think of a Bodhisattva's grace and control his eating. The harder the work, the more he may eat. When he is not working, he should eat only a small amount. Even when the opportunity comes to have rich food, he must restrict his intake and not eat too much. After practicing this way, he will not need to be engaged in physical labor very long and will be able to advance in society. There are many laborers who have climbed up in society and become prosperous. They all had humility. I have tried this method on several people with success.

The Way to Use Money and the Crossroads
of Wealth and Poverty

One who has physiognomic signs of wealth cannot be judged wealthy as long as he doesn't take good care of gold and silver. His fortune will definitely decline. Such a person would not respect his parents and ancestors and become unhappy. Gold, silver, and copper — these three items are tools to govern the country. They are an important tripod like the three teachings (Shinto, Confucianism, and Buddhism) and the three graces (master, teacher, parent). When these three — gold, silver, and copper — are lacking, we cannot see smoke from houses. When there is a shortage of 1 *sen* from 1000 *kan*, it is no longer 1000 *kan*.[16] Therefore 1 *sen* has as much virtue as 1000 *kan*. Money circulates in society endlessly for the benefit of people like the movement of yin and yang. Such work is like that of parents who take care of their children. Parental love is limitless.

Therefore, one who handles money carelessly is as bad as one who does not respect his parents' love. Money, like parents, then leaves him. Eventually, his house declines. If you want to keep gold and silver in your house, respect the virtue of money like your master and do not waste even 1 *sen*. When you have to pay others, pray in your mind for the money to return to your home again. When it comes back to you, pray in your mind as though your master has come back to stay with you for a long time.

If you handle money with such care, you will be observing the order of heaven and earth. Everything will go smoothly and even with physiognomic signs of poverty you can certainly prosper. It is easy to go visit someone who respects you. You can stay a long time. But if you go to see someone who treats you like a piece of stone tile, you don't want to stay very long. This is not only money but every phenomena, including humans. Money feels the same way, too. That is heaven's order.

Look at those who are poor or lose their wealth and home. They all handled money carelessly. Also those who are rich or come from an old established family line, you will notice how carefully they treat money. You can see this sincerity in their nature.

C. Food and Mental Illness

A person with physiognomic signs of mental illness will not develop such illness if he strictly controls his food. One with physiognomic signs of mental illness will certainly develop such illness if he eats in a disorderly way and his spirit gets disturbed by a fox.[17] Usually a person with mental craziness is too strong. This abnormally strong liver energy creates a deficiency in balance and attracts a lower spirit.[18] The treatment lies in proper food and drink. Do not argue with a mentally ill person who talks nonsense like a demon but just treat him as an ordinary person. After giving him only three meals a day without any snacks for 100 days, the fox or badger spirit will leave him automatically. Even being ill for some years, he can be naturally cured after three years of such controlled eating. The cure doesn't mean the animal spirit has left. He gets well because his liver gets quieter by strictly controlling his food and by developing his own healthy, balanced spirit. Even when a fox or badger spirit comes to someone, if his spiritual energy is healthy and balanced, it cannot interfere with him and leaves by itself. You should know any such illness is always caused by disorderly eating. When someone becomes mentally ill, people tend to give them whatever they wish to eat and drink. This is very disorderly. That's why such a person's mind becomes disturbed. His liver *ki* enormously increases and grows disorderly, and he cannot be cured. Food is the essence to nourish the mind. Therefore, if the essence is disturbed, so is the mind.

D. One who has a proper amount of food but indulges in rich gourmet food will not prosper even with physiognomic signs of success. Such a person will not gain any wealth, even with physiognomic signs of large wealth. Daily food should match our means and income. As the lord has his appropriate food, the samurai earning 10,000 *koku* has his appropriate food, the junior officer has his appropriate fare. When a person of no rank eats like someone of high rank, he will never advance. Therefore, those who indulge in sensory and rich food will never prosper, even with good physiognomy. A man of middle rank who eats like a man of low rank can extend his food to attain high rank. Therefore, those who are modest and do not indulge will progress and prosper in society. A man of middle rank who eats like a man of middle rank can achieve things appropriately.

Therefore, one will be able to progress without failure so long as he strictly limits his food to one bowl of rice and one side dish. There are some poor men who eat very simply only one side dish. This alone is fine, but they tend to eat sometimes a lot of quantity and therefore become poorer. They make themselves poor. That is why someone who becomes humble and modest, we say they create their own wealth.

E. A laborer earns good money, but because of his big eating he is accumulating a loan from heaven and earth. Therefore, he has to labor all his life. Because he has this loan from heaven and earth, he must work or otherwise run out of food. No one will lend money to a poor man who doesn't work to pay him back. The same rule applies to the relation between a man and heaven. Therefore, one who eats more than his share can never progress in life and has to continue working till the end of his life. Nevertheless, those big eaters can extend their grace to heaven and earth by being frugal. Naturally they will always have a little extra to count on, and they can be more relaxed. To prosper does not lie only in working hard in business. To prosper there is no other way but being frugal, extending the food given to us by heaven.

Beyond having enough food, clothing, and doing what you wish, it is foolish to wish to climb to a higher level in society. I can tell you again and again be moderate and respect your food.

#10 Modesty in Food and Drink Decides Personality

Monk's Food

A. Modesty in food determines whether your personality is noble or poor. Why are famous monks and wise men noble and respected? Because they are very humble, reduce their food, and refrain from a disorderly way of eating. In this way, they create their own noble personality. People will not respect even a distinguished "man of knowledge" who has a humble attitude toward other people but has no humility in eating.

B. Those who eat more than their share will have bad fortunes, find difficulties in many things, and have to face some unexpected losses. The only thing heaven has given you is a certain amount of food. When you are eating more than your share, you are creating a food debt to heaven. Wasted food becomes nothing but excrement, never directly benefiting society. When can you pay back your debt to heaven? If you borrow money from a person, he sends you a bill. But heaven doesn't send a bill. It collects your debt without asking. If you cannot pay it back, heaven collects it from your descendents. If there are no descendents, it will destroy your house and end your family tree. It's the order of heaven and earth to return what you have borrowed. Therefore, one who takes more than his share will have bad fortune and face many unexpected accidents and losses. They result simply from heaven collecting your debt through punishment.

#11 The Way to Avoid Misfortune in an Unlucky Cycle of the Year

One who has bad physiognomy in an unlucky cycle of the year can avoid any accident by not indulging in eating at all and by strictly controlling his food. One who eats a big quantity and irregularly will certainly have to face some accident in his unlucky yearly cycle. A baby up to three years old is in an unlucky phase, also adults between the age of forty-one and forty-three.[19] The latter is just beginning to be old. Therefore, he surely faces difficulties unless he is humble.

You pay back your earlier debt in the latter unlucky stage. Therefore, one who has not been humble since youth will certainly encounter misfortune. To avoid this, you must start praying three years earlier to whichever diety or Buddha you believe in as your protective diety. The proper way to pray involves reducing by half your food intake and giving this to your protective spirit. Then you can purify earlier vices you may have committed during these three years.

I do not mean you actually offer half of your food on the altar but at the table offer half in your mind by giving up the thought of wanting to eat it yourself. However small the food you prepare, you must offer half of it to the protective diety instead of eating all of it. Then there is no doubt that you can avoid misfortune.

When you pray in such a way for three years, you can change a short life into a long one and poverty into wealth. I will mention how to predict bad fortune later in this book. One who has not settled into a moderate and orderly way of eating but eats aggressively, even with good physiognomic signs of wealth, will not realize good fortune but will have to face big difficulties. The eating of such a person has not stabilized. Nor can he smoothly leave his wealth to his descendents. His aggressive eating will always injure him. By destroying his food, he destroys his wealth. Wealth is totally dependent on what you eat. Therefore, chaotic eating produces only a chaotic income. Aggressive eaters sometimes exhibit a facial color accompanying good fortune, but that color is not true. Rather it shows his arrogance. No really good face color from heaven would appear in a person who is not humble, though he might be able to achieve something small.

B. A fat person enjoying a lot of meat and sake will never prosper in society during his lifetime. Unless he becomes humble, his fortune will be bad at old age. With lots of sake and meat, your flesh becomes loose and unclear and does not correspond to your bone structure. Though he looks great, he is not a great man at all. He looks big only because he increased his blood supply from consuming so much meat and sake, but actually that makes his mind flabby, and his whole body is loose.

A man depends on the *ki* of his mind. One whose mind *ki* stays in his bones has steady energy. Therefore he will be able to manage himself well and progress by himself. There is no one in the world who can prosper with loose *ki* in himself.

C. In addition to sake or meat, overeating and rich food will make the flesh flabby and lead away from lifelong success and prosperity. After you eat rich food and your stomach becomes full, your *ki* becomes very heavy and you grow sleepy. This all results from loose mind *ki* and loose flesh. Therefore, anyone who eats more than his share creates sagging flesh and will not be able to advance in life at all. There are a few big eaters who gradually lose weight. Such people are just waiting to die of illness from wrong eating. There are some people with strong mind *ki* who do not lose weight from overeating and overdrinking. Nevertheless, they lose their good face color and progressing *ki*. Therefore thin people who overeat will never prosper.

D. There are a few people who eat more than others and still live a long life. In that case, their amount of heaven-sent food is very large. People with thick skin are always ones who have received a lot of food from heaven at birth. But even those who have such a structure, unless they are humble, will indulge in the food given to them and will not be able to live at ease throughout their life. They all will be the authors of their own destruction. By eating humbly and modestly, people with physiognomic signs showing lots of food given to them by heaven at birth will progress very well in life and attain good fortune.

#12 Eating a Little Meat in Old Age Creates Minor Ill Effects

A. It is not against the laws of nature for the very old to eat a little meat because their declining body can be nourished in this way. Nevertheless, it is very important for them to take only a reasonably very small amount. Young trees do not naturally decline, but old trees do. Meager food cannot sustain old trees. In such a case, they can be kept alive with manure or excrement as fertilizer. Therefore, the old can be nourished by food. Nevertheless, one who has been indulging in rich food from an early age will not be able to grow old. Therefore, you must be humble from the start and extend your food, in this way keeping your longevity. They you can show respect to your parents and elders.[20]

B. It is certainly wrong to like meat and sake and eat a lot of it. Such people will never enjoy longevity. Busy city persons eat rich food and animal food. Such people will develop an imbalanced mind and act aggressively. Big meat-eaters will always turn out wrong. Those who eat simple food can develop a balanced mind and avoid bad conduct. That's why there are few bad people in the countryside but many in the busy cities.

As animals, birds and fish also have life. Therefore, if you kill and eat them, you are actually taking your own life. Therefore city people tend to live short lives, and mountain people live long ones. Busy city people eat rich food and develop mental difficulties. Mountain people, on the other hand, eat simple fare and create no such difficulties. Poverty, happiness, and a long or short life all depend on food.

If one eats meat properly and in small amount, he can receive nourishment and keep longevity. In such a case, birds and fish nourish human life by being eaten. That is their happiness in life. It is a benevolent heart. Too much animal food creates sickness and destroys the eater's life. In such cases, people tend to blame the birds and fish instead of themselves. It is a sin to kill birds and fish before they have completed their life's purpose. In Buddhism, this is considered a sin against the rule of not taking life.[21] Even a monk, though, who properly eats a small amount of animal food, can nourish himself well and stay on the Buddhist path. He is not breaking the rule. But, of course, if he forgets the spirit of Buddha and eats in a disorderly way, he is breaking the rule and will become less than an ordinary man.

#13 A Child's Physiognomic Signs of Poverty or Bad Conduct Are the Responsibility of the Parents

Food and the Future of Children

A. A child with diagnostic signs of a life of poverty may not necessarily be poor as long as the parents are very humble in their practice. Bad physiognomic signs in a child can change to good ones according to the behavior of the parents. Parents are the origin of the child. If the origin is right, the child can develop properly. Even when it is a question of bad karma incurred prior to the child's birth, the parents can release such karma by their good behavior.[22] If your parents did not release such bad karma when you were small, you should do it by yourself now. Such karma can only be released by practicing yin virtue.[23]

There are some people who make donations, contribute to society, and liberate captive animals. But these are not at all yin virtue because other people recognize it. True yin virtue is to cut down a half bowl of the food you were going to eat and to offer and extend it to heaven and earth. This is true yin virtue, or hidden grace, because no one but you is aware of it.

Even at mealtime there is invisible merit in saving one mouthful of food. This can help release any bad karma you have accumulated as well as that passed on to your descendents. It is as obvious as pointing your finger at the full moon.

B. There are many people with the worst physiognomic signs who have changed themselves and become wealthy and successful by being deeply humble and frugal.[24] If you have physiognomic signs of poverty, you can attain a prosperous life by striving to be frugal.

I will give you one example. There was a man called Sumiyoshi at Dojima in Osaka with the nickname of "Fighting Yoichi." In his youth, he was a professional gambler and earned a reputation for sowing wild oats. I saw in him physiognomic signs of being violent and poor as well as ending up a cripple. Nevertheless, he was really sad to see anything wasted. He sometimes won a lot of gold and silver from gambling which he spent freely. Yet even in such cases, he would not indulge himself in drinking and eating and always liked soft rice. Many times he would come across some bamboo or wood floating down the river or which someone left lying on the ground. He collected it and made firewood. He cooked his own food and prepared a very small amount. Though he never studied anything and remained formally ignorant, naturally he accumulated wealth and later in life was very happy. By learning to extend his virtue to everything in nature, he created a good environment around him. Therefore, anyone can advance in society even with extremely bad physiognomic signs by wasting nothing and being frugal. This is the reason why talking only about physiognomy is useless. Destiny depends all on one's modesty.

C. Compulsory big eaters never fail to become unsuccessful. Even with physiognomic signs of respecting parents, one who eats a lot and in a disorderly way gets serious illnesses and eventually loses the body which his parents have given him. Dying before your parents is the worst action you can do to them.[25] One can start to respect his parents by being humble in eating, even with diagnostic signs indicating no respect to one's father and mother. There are people who teach the importance of respecting parents and who get sick through disorderly eating. Such people are ignorant. Humble eaters are approaching the Tao, even without any formal learning.

D. If you wish to be successful and advance in the future, you ought to reduce your food intake and keep practicing a humble and modest way of eating. If you practice this well, you will never fail to advance in life. Without controlling your food, you will never to able to prosper. Because one who has decided to control his eating already has a quiet and steady mind, he can control his body. He knows when to stop eating and can extend his food and will remain steady. Those who have not come near to the Tao would find difficulty in controlling their food. Being able to control one's food is the tao of a human being. It is useless to talk about people who are wandering around and just eating and drinking. Such people are like animals who eat, pass through life, and die without realizing any insight or wisdom. They are just like old men who produce feces and do not plow. There are many such foolish persons in the world.

#14 One Can Recover the Prosperity of His House by Reducing His Food

The Master of the House's Way of Eating and the House's Rise and Decline

A. Even after a wealthy house declines, when the head of the household cuts down the amount of food he eats, the house would again be able to recover and prosper.[26] The master of the family is like a god in the house. Even when the house's fortune has run out, the house will not decline with a master who is strict in his eating. Households invariably declined because the master indulged. When the fortune of the house has run out, it means the house has exhausted the food given to it by heaven, and the house runs out of wealth. When the house runs out of food and wealth, the house will certainly decline. Therefore, if a master of the household reduces his food and extends the food he has saved, the wealth of the house will also be extended. With enough food and wealth, a house will never decline.

B. One who recognizes his physiognomic signs of poverty will certainly be able to gain gold and silver by strictly controlling his way of eating and taking simple food. This is self-made happiness and grace. When you are poor, live as a poor man. Then prosperity comes to you by itself. But a poor man who feels sad and yearns for prosperity, decorating only the outside, will certainly lose his grace and become even poorer. Therefore, you must be virtuous to heaven and earth instead of trying to be wealthy. Then prosperity and grace come to you by themselves.

No one with physiognomic signs of poverty will become poor so long as he reduces his food and practices well. Real poverty comes only to those who indulge in food and drink. They have made themselves poor. Nevertheless, when you reduce the amount of food you eat, it is not too bad to include lots of grains and vegetables. The standard of simple eating is one bowl of rice and one side dish.

C. One who wants to advance in some tao, as well as succeed in his profession as a samurai, farmer, craftsman, or merchant, should be modest in eating and keep his distance from women. But after his training is completed, he may enjoy their company. Even then, he should not have one who is disobedient and who does not follow the tao. Such a woman will certainly injure his reputation and disturb his training. Even a foolish man and a man with a small personality can understand natural order, but a woman does not. Be extra careful. One who has difficulty in finding a wife is a man who can advance well in some tao. Such a person should master the tao for other people and regard his attainment as his offspring so that he can still honor his parents. Then your spirit will never disappear.

The Way to Use Water and Fire for Longevity

D. One with physiognomic signs of longevity cannot live long if he wastes water. If he continues to live, he will become poorer and more unfortunate and probably end up without any children. No one can attain longevity if he wastes oil and enjoys a big, bright light. If you are very careful in using water and light, you will certainly maintain longevity and happiness. Water corresponds to the kidneys in the body. Therefore, one who wastes water hurts his kidneys' spirit. Weak kidneys only injure his lifespan, and he cannot live long. Also water produces trees and is the beginning of nourishment for all living things. When one hurts this essence, he naturally cannot nourish himself and produce a child. Even if he has a child, he will certainly become poorer. If you extend your life and attain happiness, first be careful when you handle water. One who uses light or fire too brightly is very excitable. Therefore, one who has deficient kidneys dislikes darkness and becomes even more deficient with more light.

The Way to Use Paper and Yin Virtue

E. One with physiognomic signs of prosperity will not be able to be prosperous so long as he wastes paper. The same applies for those with signs of virtue. If such a person is poor, he will remain in poverty his whole life and cannot manage anything. Paper is made with a lot of water. Since ancient times, they say a piece of paper is made with one *to* of water. When such is the case, paper is a diety — righteous and clear.[28]

When you put your seal or stamp on a piece of paper that shows your sincerity and makes things clear.[29] One who wastes paper certainly hurts his grace and will attract poverty all his life and be unable to manage. Cheap paper is made with a little water. Therefore, one cannot be blamed for using it to blow his nose or for going to the toilet. Nothing is wrong with using white paper if properly used. Only when one uses it carelessly does he hurt his grace. A careless person uses white paper to blow his nose and in the toilet. One who has some humility uses white paper four to five times before using it as toilet paper. A very humble person would save the used toilet paper and give it to papermakers for recycling. This is yin virtue. Once thrown into a toilet, the paper can never be recovered. There are no papermakers in the countryside or in the mountains where eventually white paper may have to be wasted. Nevertheless, everyone should remember to recycle paper and practice yin virtue.

F. If you don't take care of your tools and new possessions and respect them as they become older, we can't say that you have a really good, honest heart. You should respect them as your servants. If you take care of them only when they are new but throw them away when they are old, your attitude is not right. You should return old china and earthenware to the soil and burn things made of wood and return their ashes to the earth. This is like the mercy of a lord who attends to his minister's death. Such careful persons, even if their physiognomy is not so good, are honest and sincere. However you manage things day to day shows the physiognomy of your life and reveals your destiny. A person's physiognomic signs appear in everything in the world. Therefore it is not enough just to discuss facial structure and other superficial features.

#15 One with Good Physiognomic Signs Cannot Advance in Society If He Likes Playing *Go* or *Shogi*

A. If your physiognomic structure is very good but you like playing *go* or *shogi*, you cannot climb up in society.[30] The exception is those who are professionals in the game. Playing *go* and *shogi* brings bad fortune to ordinary people who have to take care of themselves and their household. Those who like these pastimes cannot manage things well around them. Games yield only brief enjoyment. One who really wants to succeed doesn't think of such things. Without wasting their energy on such pursuits, they concentrate on what is really important in life and eventually they reach their goal with the aid of heaven. Even just a short time playing around can weaken your vision and reduce your energy. It is very bad. But when you put all your *ki* into your business or job, you work very hard and never forget your dream. But because games and pastimes are so enjoyable, you completely forget yourself and enjoy only the moment. If you really wish to accomplish something in life, refrain from games and pastimes.

#16 A House with a Nice Garden of Small Mountains and Fountains Will Decline

A house with a beautiful garden of small mountains and fountains cannot progress, even with geomantic signs of good fortune.[31] It can only decline. Having and enjoying such a garden which imitates real mountains and seas is only for people who have a very high position and great wealth. Therefore, when an ordinary person enjoys like someone with high rank and wealth, he must be overindulging in life. He will never advance. Even a wealthy family with such a garden can never flourish. Sometimes if the grace received from ancestors is great and the house is flourishing, a family with such a garden may not decline but it won't prosper. There are many such cases. Try to find some. Such a house has sick persons frequently. Therefore, if a person with a beautiful garden wants to advance his house, he must replace it with a shrine to whatever religion he believes in, pray to God or Buddha, and give away food to the poor. Then the house will prosper. Even in such a case, you cannot gain anything if you eat as much as you wish and set aside food offerings to the deity. Pray for the prosperity of the house by offering the food you were going to have.

B. One with physiognomic signs of advancement who enjoys a gorgeous flowerbed will never progress. That is only for people of high rank. Therefore, such a person will hurt the grace sent to him from heaven and earth and will not be able to achieve anything in life. In the case of a wealthy family where a person of high rank may visit from time to time, they may have such a flowerbed, but it should not be for their own enjoyment. The earth is the mother of everything. When you sow seeds, they grow. If you have a reasonably sized garden, you must grow grains and vegetables. Such a garden accumulates grace from heaven and earth. The meeting of heaven's energy and earth's energy produces plants which nourish men. When a man helps to grow the plant, his virtue increases. One who does not understand virtue and indulges in enjoyment will naturally violate his grace and be unable to progress. There are those who have a good time growing edible plants as nice as a flowerbed. I have seen such people all advance in society and their houses prosper with grace from heaven and earth.

The Way to Use Fire for Success

C. There are a few people with good physiognomy who start fire without any purpose or carelessly step on it to put it out. Such people will never advance in their whole life and cannot manage anything. *Fire* is also *day*.[32] Therefore, careless stepping on fire is like stepping on the sun, the universal emperor. Fire is also important for warmth. Without fire, even for a day, it is difficult to sustain one's life. If you waste fire, which warms things up, you will never be hot at anything and be unable to manage things. Yang fire has a quality of good fortune. If you handle fire carelessly and disorderly, you will lose good fortune. Most people who are not humble in their food also do not respect fire. They face many troubles.

D. One who is steady and strict in his way of eating will have good face color and God will appear in him. God will not appear in those who eat aggressively and disorderly. Someone filled with God will maintain steady face color. His appearance or expression will not change. But someone who lacks God in himself will have an unsteady face color. And one who is not modest tends to change appearance and expression often. His good fortune easily changes to misfortune. One who is modest and strict in eating has firm flesh which becomes well balanced and taut with his bones. It is wrong to call such a person skinny. His spirit is very fat or rich. God shines through his appearance and expression.

But if one overeats without any control, his *ki* becomes heavy and skinny. In such a case, God does not shine through him. His heart, liver, and lungs become overactive. Then his spleen, pancreas, and kidneys get weak and then his muscles and flesh deteriorate. This is true skinniness — inner weakening of *ki* — as shown by a slight dark color all over the body.

A humble person with good tight flesh and bones looks skinny but will have opaque skin without any faint darkness. This method shows how to judge if someone is declining or not. You must be able to recognize rich or fat *ki* in a skinny person. What a sorry feeling to have a declining body.

Book II

A. Managing Your Body through Spiritual Control

Q. I wanted to become an expert in some cultural or spiritual tao. I have tried many times and put my whole heart and soul into this. But my wife and child are always disturbing me. My wife is a bad woman. She is always hen-pecking, criticizing, and making difficulties. As a result my study does not go far. What shall I do?

A. If you are a big man with a great capacity — but even if you are an ordinary man — wanting to excel in any tao, it is better not to marry. You have to really concentrate on your tao or path in life. If your spirit becomes sincere and strong like the sun, small yin won't disturb you, and you can achieve the tao. But if you are not like the great sun — not strong of heart — you will attract a wife who is very yin. That's why you have attracted many difficulties and are stuck. We say man is yang and woman is yin. If the wife doesn't follow the yang husband, yin and yang don't match well. If yang and yin don't complement each other well, then your tao will never be accomplished. If your wife doesn't follow you, you can't accomplish your dream in society and people won't listen to you. We can say it another way: if your wife doesn't follow you, then naturally society won't follow your path or listen to your teachings.

B. The Wife Is the Treasure of the House

Whether you are a samurai, farmer, carpenter, engineer, or merchant, if your wife is good, then everything naturally turns out well and the family becomes prosperous. A disorderly house is caused by the wife. She is the treasure of the house. If that treasure is bad, the house will cease to exist.[1] The wife occupies the governing place in the family and is called "governor." [2] The wife is yin. That's why her (yin) position is in the north. The husband is south and yang, and she follows her husband.[3] The wife is called "a person in the north." [4] This is the family's heart, the central tree. A person in the north (wife) is the base of all growth, following a person in the south (husband). Therefore, she is called "the respectful base place." [5] She is also called "a person at the deep back." [6] Because she is always following her husband, we use that respectful name. If the wife is not good, that is, not a treasure, she becomes a demon and destroys the house. That's why the husband can't achieve his tao. Buddha once said, "If someone is a great man, demons always come as his wife, child, or friend disturbs his way." Such a bad wife may be a demon. You have to escape or get away from her. If you can't leave quickly, she will disturb your way and reputation. The *Heart Sutra* says, "If a devil bothers you, leave it behind, and it will become like a deity and protect you." [7] If you leave her, she may change to a good heart and follow you. At that time you can marry again. If you have a child and leave a devilish wife, that is a great mistake. In my own case, I really wish to spread my teachings for many years, but it's very difficult to be successful. I have a foolish wife like yours, so I have great difficulties. Even saints have difficulties like this.

#2 The Origin of All Good and Bad Things Is Food

A. Food and Fortune and Misfortune

Q. Sensei, you talk only about strictly eating and drinking and not about fortune and misfortune. You don't talk about physiognomy. A proverb says, "Too much is just like not enough." [8] Please read ancient texts and talk more about physiognomy and fortune-telling.

A. I sincerely listen to you. From an early age, my parents were very poor. That's why I didn't read or write and could not read any books. Later I listened to a teacher of classical physiognomy, but for just a few days. Also I was not so interested in following the old masters. But three years ago, among my disciples, there was a scholar. He read to me Confucius's book, *The Great Way of Governing the World*. At that time I was forty-seven. For the first time in my life I heard his wonderful teachings. I clearly understood the bright value of physiognomy. Real physiognomy is a great tao to maintain one's health and guide society and the world. That's why I'm gathering many ordinary people and explaining to them my way of life. With that in mind, I started talking to them about fortune and misfortune. But recently, I'm just guiding people and not talking so much about fortune and misfortune. I have discovered that food alone is the real origin and beginning of this way of life. That's why I'm talking so much about food and drink.[9] Everything I am saying is for the purpose of managing your heart, spirit, and body. I can truly say that soul and body are nourished by food. If your food and drink are not steady and strong, you cannot manage your mind and body. That's why food is important. Your happiness comes from food. Your sadness comes from food. Everything — millions of good and bad things — are all caused by food.[10]

B. Yin Virtue and Releasing Life

Q. I sincerely ask you, you are always talking about yin and yang and about grace. I understand yin grace is when your donation remains hidden. Yang grace is when it becomes known to other people. But I am confused which is better. Is it right to give money and things to other people if they take notice?

A. If you expect some kind of return from your donation, that is departing from the way. It is a mistake. If you are born, you die. If you wish to kill someone, then you can kill him. It is really not your fault. The same way, if you wish to help other people, you can help them. But that action doesn't necessarily carry good merit. Birth and death all come from heaven. Sometimes you wish to help, but you kill as a result. Who is to be blamed? The fault's within. Or you may wish to kill someone, but actually you help them. Those things do not constitute virtue. Whatever you want to do originates from heaven. You may think that you have donated or given away something, but what really are you able to give? Fortune and money belong to heaven, not to you. Even the food you give belongs to heaven which governs everyone. Where am I from? Where do I get what I donate? The only thing that belongs to you is the daily food you require to keep alive. If you give away your own food, that is real yin virtue. But if you eat to your heart's content and then give away surplus food to other people, there is no merit in that.

If you cut down the quantity of food you eat and give it away to others, that is true donation. Don't eat to capacity. If you observe this rule, you are called a man of yin virtue, and your virtue will accumulate everywhere in heaven and earth. Such a person, even if his life is short, will be very happy. Even if he is poor, he still will be rich. Countless accidents and misfortunes can be avoided in this way. Such a person will never have enemies in any direction.

In our society there is a society known as *Ho-Jo*, the Releasing Life Club.[11] This association collects live birds and fish and releases them after Buddhist monks read to them from the *Dhyani Sutra*.[12] Such practices are not really harmonizing with the order of nature. The Emperor may do such things, but for ordinary people it is not meritorious. It really doesn't help the fishermen. I have watched what happens to the birds and fish after they are released. The animals are confused and disoriented because they are often brought a far distance. It's like a disabled man from the countryside taken to Kyoto and left in a busy street.[13] You would be confused too. But that is just what they are doing. Also they are collecting the kind of animals people are eating for food. They aren't collecting mice and snakes.

Not eating birds and fish every day, that is true *ho-jo*. Or suppose we think about rice. If we put one grain in the soil, one thousand grains will be produced by the end of the year. If we sow one cup[14] of grain, one thousand cups will return. This year one thousand cups, next year one million, the year after that one billion, and so on. If every day you save one cupful of rice from your daily food, that means three years later you will accumulate a billion cups of rice. By cutting back in your food, you are practicing *ho-jo* every day. The same with carp and trout. If you think about it, one carp has millions of eggs. Three years later, we can't even calculate the number of offspring. That's why reducing the quantity of your daily food is true *ho-jo*, real donation.

C. The Way of Animals and a Man of Animals

Q. I sincerely ask you, Sensei, you talk only about food and say that if we are humble and modest our supply of food is always enough. But if we don't eat enough, we are always unsatisfied, just like the way of hungry ghosts.[15] What do you think?

A. Of course, food is to sustain life. Nevertheless, if we eat too much and in a disorderly way, we will die just like trees and grasses that receive too much fertilizer. People who destroy their life because of bad eating are just like this. If you are very humble and modest about food, you will prosper like grasses and trees. Your life will become whole, and you will be able to grow. If you are a big eater and love gourmet food, you are shooting an arrow at yourself. Your spirit is greedy. We call such a greedy person who is always eating an animal demon. Their face is human, but their heart is animal. Animals with four legs desire to run around day and night and indulge in food. You look like a human, but your body is an animal's.

Once after listening to my talk about the humble way of eating, someone asked me why I wasn't eating like other people but taking just a very small amount of barley and soba. He said it looked like I was born a hungry ghost and asked if I felt sad about this. Though he didn't know his limitations, and I knew he couldn't comprehend what I said, I replied to other people in the group: Number 1, even the Emperor and Shogun's main food is rice. The common people are also eating rice. Doesn't this frighten you? You are eating rice three times a day, and yet you are not really satisfied. If you eat wheat instead of rice, you feel like you're a hungry ghost.[16] If you think that way, you don't really know what you are. Barley is precious after rice. There are many classes of people. The byproduct of tofu should be more than enough for very low grade persons like us.[17] Even that is too rich for our walk of life. But still we are eating barley and refined rice every day.[18] We really have to give great thanks for that. Please understand this order for your happiness when departing for the next world. Please eat barley and humble yourself. We should really be thankful and modest when it comes to food.

D. **Q. I am a big bird, not a sparrow. I am not satisfied with sparrow's food. What do you advise?**

A. A big bird and sparrow — each has its limitations and the right amount and quality of food. You belong to the sparrow group. A roc doesn't eat to full capacity and is not disorderly.[19] A phoenix, another big bird, lives on mainly cold water.[20] A little bird eats anything from rice, insects, and nuts to even the excrement of horses, cows, and people. A little bird doesn't care how much it eats. You are just like this. You eat lots, just like a very disorderly sparrow, anything warm or cold until you feel full. You cannot become a sage. But your speech is like a roc's, your mind is like a sparrow's, and your appetite is like a crow's. What a unique structure and personality you have. You are a rare bird indeed! The characters of three different birds are in you.

D. The Difference Between Health and Looking Strong

Q. I am very ambitious. That's why I'm eating rich food and drinking sake. I take it to nourish my body and mind and go out into society and accomplish something. If I eat modestly, my energy weakens, and it's difficult to do anything. Is this not appropriate?

A. Healthy energy comes from heaven. This leads to happiness and joy. Automatically you become fulfilled. Real vitality is not merely physical strength or aggressiveness. You cannot acquire real vitality by eating more food. Nowadays people of so-called health and strength are nothing more than aggressive. Indulging with meat and sake is not the way of human beings. There are a few such people who successfully climb up the ladder in society. But such a person is attempting something beyond their limitation. Their actions do not correspond with heaven's order, so they can never sustain their position very long. On the other hand, if someone is very humble in their way of eating and climbs up in society and prospers, they can sustain their position a long time.

You say that you have always desired to become prosperous and advance in life. You wish it only in your mind, but don't practice it in diet. If you are modest and humble, then you will really become successful. If you cultivate the modesty of ordinary people, you can achieve only ordinary success. If you are humble beyond that, you can enjoy greater success and promotion than ordinary people. If you are the most humble person in thousands of people, you will be able to attain the success of thousands. Food nourishes your body and mind and is the origin of the greatest humility. That's why ordinary people find it difficult to be humble in food. Proper eating is the hardest thing in life. If you can be modest in your way of eating, you can far surpass the success of ordinary people. Just concentrate on a simple, grateful way of eating, and you will succeed.

#3 Why Shinto Priests Are Usually Poor and Buddhist Monks Rich.

A. **Q. I've noticed that even in famous Shinto shrines, rich priests are very rare. But in Buddhist temples, monks are usually very rich and sometimes have money to loan to people. How do you account for this?** [21]

A. Shinto is yang, and its spirit is aggressive, strong, and very clean. Running water never becomes stagnant. Cleansing doesn't lead to accumulation. Shinto priests lay great emphasis on purity and are pure themselves but poor. On the other hand, Buddhism is yin. Its spirit is quiet and relaxed. Buddhist monks don't mind dirt and dust. Naturally, many things come and accumulate in their temples, and they become rich.

Among modern day Buddhists, there are some who have chaotic thinking but don't eat meat. No monks seek eroticism or wives and children. They keep modesty and observe their rules, but naturally their desires are not fulfilled. Because of this modesty and refraining from indulgence, heaven and earth sustain them and bestow grace in the form of wealth. Though poor materially, they enjoy good fortune. This is the natural order of wealth.

Shinto priests have wives and children and often drink sake, eat meat, and seek for pleasures. Eventually their grace runs out, and there is a big breakdown. That's why even famous shrines become poor according to the order of heaven. I don't know about upper class people, but in the case of lower class people, if we are not modest, we shall be unsuccessful. That is heaven's order. Whether high or low, noble or peasant, if they please as they like every day and ignore their limitations, they will never be able to realize their tao.

B. Achieving Happiness, Wealth and Longevity with Food

Q. I would like to progress and attain happiness, wealth, and longevity. If I am more humble and modest, can I accomplish this or not?

A. Progress to achieve happiness, wealth, and longevity comes from a humble food pattern. If your determination is very strong, naturally you restrict your food, too. Food is just like your mind, also like your emperor. Wealth, long life, and happiness are hence their ministers. Food is just like an emperor. If your food is chaotic, then your wealth, long life, and happiness cannot be achieved like a country that becomes chaotic and war arises from a chaotic emperor and ministers. If the king is good, then the country and nation will not become chaotic. The three ministers — wealth, long life, and happiness — are loyal and keep everything in good condition under such a good emperor.

We can also look at it another way. If you want to achieve these three ends, don't seek only pleasure. What are your limits? You must know them. You must know what you really need and what you can do without. You should understand the boundaries to your desire. If you are very modest and humble and unfulfilled, heaven will fill you with satisfaction. That is the order of nature. The realization of happiness, wealth, and longevity, as well as prosperity and success, depends entirely on how much you eat, how much you spend, and how much you save.

Because money belongs to society, even if you spend it, it always exists somewhere and never stops circulating. If you eat one extra bowl of rice, the surplus goes into your excrement. You lose grace. If you are chaotic and eat plenty of food, you will naturally lose your life, health, and happiness. Someone who destroys those things does so only by food. All difficulties arise from nothing but a chaotic way of eating. Do not eat much and extend what you have. In this way, you can accumulate grace every day and become prosperous later on.

Because you were modest, the food you saved daily eventually fills the whole of heaven and earth, and you will become successful in society. The virtue you have created will return to you as prosperity. Fortune or misfortune does not depend upon your physiognomic structure. Please be modest in eating.

C. The True Meaning of Eating Animal Food and Getting Married

Q. In the Honganji sect of Jodo Shin Shu Buddhism, the priests marry and even eat animal food.[22] They look strong and aggressive, but still they are very rich. And their life ends with wealth. Why?

A. Ignorance, especially that of ordinary people in society, is difficult to overcome. If priests who are very pure and clean try to guide them, ordinary people are usually too afraid to come near. If they won't approach you, you can't talk to or preach to them. That's why the founder of Jodo Shin Shu, with his grace, changed the outward appearance of his sect to ordinary people.[23] People look at the priests' behavior and automatically feel comfortable. Naturally they come to the temple and gather to follow the Buddha Way. Then they clean up their illusion or ignorance. This is the greatest yin virtue. Because of this approach, the Jodo Shin Shu sect has became very popular, and naturally the priests became rich. In this case, the priests marry and eat animal food from a great mercy. They are truly worshipping the Buddha. But sometimes the monks of this sect don't understand the founder's real heart and intention and just indulge, marry, and eat animal food for pleasure. Those type of monks are just like mice living in a food warehouse. This is natural order. They should really try to understand their founder's intention and partake of the blessing of his virtue with fear and trembling.

D. Poverty Makes Wealth and Happiness

Q. From a young age, I enjoyed great success and was very rich. But recently my destiny has turned very bad. Year by year I'm losing a lot of money. Whatever I start turns into a failure.

A. When you are young, you were very rich and your life was full. That's why now you are in decline. That is the natural order. If you fall quickly, you should think that is your great good fortune. If you don't decline of your own accord, then nature will make you decline unwillingly. If nature makes you decline, your suffering will be much greater. If you take responsibility for your own decline, it is easier and less difficult. You don't suffer so much. You can then become full again. From your physiognomy, I can see that you were originally very poor but strong and independent. You created your wealth by yourself. You should now return to your origin. Because you became arrogant and forgot what it was like to be poor, heaven sent you difficulties. If you forget your origin and beginning, you will lose everything at the end.

If someone always remembers their origin and beginnings, they will never become arrogant and never decline. Also I can say a great person is someone who has known both great happiness and wealth and great difficulties and poverty. We call this understanding the origin of life. A happy, prosperous person who understands and cares for the poor knows the beginning and end of all things. He never declines. Such a person is observing the way of humanity. They treat their servants like great kings or wonderful emperors. Their family continues because they understand the way of humanity. Wealth and blessings from the ten directions gather around them, and naturally they prosper.

Poverty is the origin of wealth. The origin of wealth and nobility is poverty. The beginning of everything is poverty. Even the emperor wasn't a king from the beginning by himself. Only when his people gathered and recognized him as emperor was he truly king. Master and subordinates depend on each other. The more subordinates gather, the higher and greater the master's position becomes. If you know poverty and know how to treat your subordinates, automatically you will become rich. If you treat your subordinates like your own children, emperor and subordinates will become one. This is the true meaning of wealth and nobility.

You should always take care of your subordinates just like a younger sister. Care for them just like your own children when they become sick. Feed them three times a day and don't make any distinction between the food they eat and the food you eat. And even if you are determined not to drink sake, two or three times a month drink sake to entertain the subordinates. Then domestic and family prosperity will follow. Don't waste or throw away things necessary for your job, but don't scold your subordinates even if they waste something. For your part, the tiniest amount of conscientiousness will save a million things from waste, especially if your way of eating is very strict. In addition to regular meals, you may give extra food to your servants but don't eat extra food yourself. If you do this for three years, your family will prosper and your house will become even richer than before. That is as sure as striking the ground with your hand.

E. The Origin of Poverty, Difficulties, and Many Sicknesses

Q. Recently I experienced many sicknesses and troubles. Gradually I am suffering more and more and becoming poorer. My family and relatives are very rich, but no one helps or takes care of me. What do you advise?

A. Depending on other people is not right. Because of your own behavior, fortune or misfortune arises. It doesn't depend on what other people do. Society and many people help and take care of you in many ways. We should be more than grateful to the Emperor who is always praying to safeguard or protect our happiness. The samurai are protecting us in the event someone wants to rob or kill us. The farmers are growing the five grains for us to eat. The carpenters and mechanics are making daily tools for us to use in our work. The merchants are stocking goods, allowing us to buy what we need. From the Emperor down to ordinary people, everyone is helping you.

Therefore, if you waste things and time, grow lazy, and are disorderly and chaotic in your way of eating without any modesty, all your organs will decay and you will become sick, even with good physiognomy. You will continue to sink into poverty. You didn't understand heaven and earth's grace and didn't control yourself. The big sicknesses and poverty that you experience do not come from birth but were created by you later. You cannot blame others. Nor is it punishment from heaven. If you are modest, cut down the quantity of food you eat, and make yourself humble. Then naturally you will become rich and cure your sickness.

#4 By Eating Humbly People Can Enjoy Some Pleasures

A man came and sincerely asked:

Q. I find it very easy to be modest in my way of eating but very difficult to be strict about playing around and spending money. What shall I do?

A. That's all right. Modesty applies primarily to food. If you go to a tavern or gambling hall and are foolishly spending money, you will not get sick and your family won't collapse so long as you remain humble and modest in your food pattern. You can still enjoy long life and remain rich. Food is really the origin or trunk. Other things are like branches. If the trunk is good, we don't even need to talk about them. Please stay humble and strict about your food. Then you can go and play if you like. You will escape from unhappiness and misfortune through modest food. Of course, there is a difference among people. Some are big, others are small. Some are strong, others are weak. But if we take the norm at three meals a day, if you are modest you will eat only 2 1/2 meals a day. And don't eat between meals. If you don't eat rich food except dried fish, then you can play around and enjoy yourself.

B. Your Job and Food Modesty

Q. If we are very humble about food and eat strictly but do not look often at our business, will we climb up in society and prosper? But doesn't success also depend on how hard we work? Please talk more about work itself.

A. Of course, starting from the Emperor down, life is accompanied by food and by work. Even animals and birds are running around, putting their energy into obtaining food. Everyone automatically has, or is given, food and work. As human beings, everyone is working in some way or another. If you aren't working, you are worse than the birds and animals. A person who does not work tends to enjoy drinking and eating animal food and their mind becomes chaotic, lazy, and they can't work. Of course, their food is too much. Therefore, they don't feel very good and can't work the following day either. Day by day, this pattern is repeated. At the end, sickness results. Everything results from not being modest in food. Modesty, strictness, and control of food is primary. Strict food makes a disciplined mind or heart. If your mind is focused, people won't push you to do anything. Food is most important.

C. Reason for Sumo Wrestlers' and Actors' Fame

Q. Sumo wrestlers are not so humble. They are arrogant in their behavior and expression. Yet they are very famous and end their lives honored by society. I wonder why this is?

A. Strong sumo wrestlers become famous across Japan because of stronger vitality than ordinary people. Their names become well known. Also there are many artists and performers who come from the lower classes but whose art is really superior. They are strong and gifted. Then they become famous. Such persons entertain people's sentimental pleasures only and are not really helping society itself. They appeal to society and are famous in their lifetime. But thirty years after they die, nobody remembers their name. But if you are modest, humble, and help many people and society itself, your fame or name will last many generations and not change. Ordinary people will feel your virtue and you will be remembered for many generations to come. This is truly working for the good of society.

D. If You Enjoy Rich Food You'll Become Poor.

Q. The mouth is for food. If you restrict what you want to eat, then you don't enjoy life. The most enjoyment in life comes from eating. It can't compare with other joys. Isn't this so?

A. There are millions of differences among people. A samurai's happiness is to attain to the top rank. A farmer's happiness is to put his whole effort into making his rice fields more productive than his ancestors. Technical workers enjoy achieving higher skills than their co-workers. A merchant finds enjoyment in striving to build up his business and get very rich. If you don't have such work or dream in life, you consider eating food your greatest joy. But if you enjoy rich food, at the end you will become very poor and never succeed. I recommend that first you become successful in life. Then you may enjoy your food. If you enjoy beautiful dishes from the beginning, heaven will give you poverty, difficulties, and misery.

You say the mouth is for food. I say it is the entrance to the toilet. What you vomit has as bad odor as stools. If you eat extra, it's the same as throwing your food in the toilet. If you still can't be disciplined, carry one cup of rice and throw it on your feces. Even if you are very bad — your face is human but your mind and heart is that of an animal — you will hesitate to throw fresh food onto excrement. Yet by eating too much, you are doing exactly that. You should be very fearful. Filling your stomach with rich food shortens your life. Nobles and rich people who eat food like this generally don't enjoy long life. Many poor people live long. Rich food makes life short, and simple food makes life long.

E. The Appearance of Animals in the Daytime and Fortune and Misfortune

Q. Mice aren't afraid of the family, and many times show up in daytime and mess around. Is this a sign of good or bad fortune?

A. Mice are yin among animals and should be active at night. It is very bad fortune for them to show up during the day. That means your house is not orderly. It is a sign that some difficulties or accidents will occur or your house will be destroyed. If the *ki* of your household is really strong and full, that is, very yang, yin animals such as mice won't appear in the daytime. If the *ki* of your house and family is very low or disappears, that is, very yin, then yin animals don't hesitate to come out in the daytime and make a mess. When the house is in decline, yang *ki* disappears, while yin *ki* increases. Then yin animals can mess around the house.

The origin of family decline lies with the head of the household. To strengthen yourself and your house, every morning and evening light candles in front of the family altar in your house and pray to Buddha and God. Then cut down the amount of your own food. After that every day give the food that you saved to the poor. Do like this strictly. Then whatever your job is, work hard, eat simply, and put your whole effort into thinking what is best for the family tomorrow. Before 4 a.m., wake up, face east, and honor the sun. From the sun you will get yang progressing energy, and the entire family will become very harmonious.

If you have an employee, he will become very devoted and follow you from the heart.[24] Also when you get up, get up before the employees do. If you don't really have a good heart, you will enjoy yourself, stay up late for pleasure, and disturb your employees' rest. Then you're eating lots of rich food, and your wife becomes too hard and mean with the workers in the house, treating them like bamboo or other objects to be used. They will not become harmonious, and you will end up destroying your house. The master is the center of the household, and the workers are at the periphery. They are just like the shadow of the master. Master and subordinates should be like body and shadow. There should be no difference in the food they eat. The master should enjoy things with his employees. When the master suffers or is sad, the employees will gladly take care of him.

This is heaven's clear, natural order. Everything depends entirely on you. That's the origin. If you don't understand this order, you are not a real master, and then the employee doesn't understand either. If the head of the household doesn't have sympathy and love, then the employee won't have them either. The employee's fortune or misfortune depends on the master's behavior. Everything happens like this. It is useless to talk about happiness and unhappiness from observing only signs of physiognomy and fortune-telling. Happiness is up to you. This is the essence of my physiognomy. Please return to a more modest and humble way of life.

#5 How to Realize Your Prayers for God

A. How to Think about Food for Worshipping God

Q. I sincerely come to see you and ask: I have not enjoyed good fortune in life. I'm really suffering. I've de-

cided to pray to God. Does it satisfy my life?

A. It's very bad. Where is God? God is everywhere and in everything. Therefore, if you really wish to do things, anything can be realized according to your wish. Even if you worship God for a thousand days and a thousand nights, unless you put your true heart into it, God cannot do anything. If you really wish to pray whole-heartedly, then give your life itself to worship God. Food is the root to nourish your life. If you give that food to God that is the same as giving away your life. Usually I say that if the usual diet consists of three bowls of food a day, you should eat two bowls and give one bowl to God. It is not necessary to worship in another way. Just sit down at table and pray with your mind and heart to God or Buddha, saying that you will eat only two bowls and save one bowl for God. Then He immediately receives the bowl you have saved. There is a proverb: "God comes to an honest person's mind." God wouldn't accept an impure spirit. But if you eat plenty or give God rich food, He is not happy and won't accept it. If you have three bowls, eat only two. Give one to God. Any kind of food, even meat and animal food, you can give to God in this way. If you do like this, anything without exception can be realized. Small wishes take one to two years to come true, while big ones might take ten years. If you worship God or Buddha like this, you will realize what you pray for.

Let me give you an example. On Inubo Mountain in Senshu county was a temple with a Fudoson statue which was spiritually very powerful.[25] Once during a holiday, a servant went down to the village to get sake for the temple on top of the mountain. On the way back from village, he stopped to take a drink. He first offered in his mind some sake to this statue, placed some on a rock, and then drunk some for himself. He brought back only a small amount left to the temple. The master of the temple was very angry. There was not enough sake for the usual religious observances. The master of the temple went to the temple to cleanse himself and pray to the Buddha. Suddenly there came a voice from heaven. "Do not worry, I already received sake on the rock." God and Buddha receive one's intention, not the actual material.

#6 Donate Part of Your Portion. That Is Real Unknown Hidden Virtue

A man came and sincerely asked.

Q. **Sensei, you teach that everyday we should accumulate hidden unknown virtue and worship God with a peaceful mind. Please give to me more details.**

A. That's good. Every day whatever you have in your rice bowl is what becomes your stool. But if you set aside just a small amount of that to God and give it to anyone who comes, you are accumulating real unrecognized virtue. God and Buddha will be very happy. They are even happy to receive animal food. What would you gain by eating the last mouthful? When you give it away instead, it is furthering the great love and grace of God or Buddha. Giving away food that is not part of your own portion is a vice. Donating only a part of what you would normally eat yourself really counts. If you do this, it doesn't matter whether you worship before a shrine or temple. God or Buddha will protect you.

I can also tell you this. A most sincere person would eat only half of his food and give away the rest. Then his stomach would become very peaceful, his *ki* energy won't stagnate, and he won't get sick. If you practice this three times a day, you can save one cup of yin virtue a day.[26] In a year's time, you will accumulate 360 cups of yin virtue and in ten years 3600 cups. In this way you will extend your virture and realize all your dreams. On this foundation, you can build your future happiness and success. If you don't extend your virtue by yourself, heaven would not give you wealth nor happiness.

B. The Five Grains Fall Down But We Don't Pick Up

Q. **Taking good care of the five grains, but leaving the ones fallen to the ground, is yin virtue. But if one grain is lost during the harvest, do we lose heaven's grace by not picking it up?**

A. Even if you are very careful at harvest time, sometimes grain will be lost to the ground. Grain that has fallen down may still nourish someone else who passes by and picks it up. Grain naturally falls down to take care of nature, just like the many birds who naturally receive their food from heaven. Humans who eat in a disorderly way — whatever they like — are no better than birds. Rich food is for upper class people. Pure, simple food is food for low class, ordinary people. If you're an ordinary low class person and eat rich food, your tastes and way of life don't match. If you're greedy for the food of upper class people, eventually your grace will end. You will eat it up. You will have nothing left to eat. There is an old proverb, "A greedy, aggressive person doesn't live long." This is natural order.

7. What Happens to a Low-Class Person Who Is Very Friendly with a High Class Person?

Q. My physiognomy indicates success, but I am still very poor and have not achieved any success. I am a merchant and spend most of my time dealing with rich people and friends in high society. I have many such connections but success still eludes me. What do you advise?

A. Even if your physiognomy suggests riches, you will never be successful your whole life if you maintain contact with high society. If you are a small person and make friends with people in high society, it will bring great chaos into your life and endanger your grace. You have to be very careful and frightened of this. Once you make contact with people at the top like that, then your life has reached a peak. It is against the order of nature to reach the top without your own efforts. If in the past, you accumulated some virtue on your own accord, you may become famous and may become friends with high society. In this case, don't worry. But if you have not accomplished something to bring you such accolade and are just getting ahead by being easy-going and friendly with upper class people, you are acting against heaven's order.

If you really wish to become successful, put an end to such friendly contact with people above you, but associate with the rich with honesty while at the same time extending your mercy and love to lower class people. Always be aware of your limitations, and don't be arrogant in your way of life. If you change and take this approach, you will become successful and realize the good fortune promised by your physiognomy. I can say that the rich may be respecting you, and it is not real respect, only because you have connections with high society and their influence and you are powerful. You have to beware of someone who wants to become friendly with you. They may be coming just to take advantage of your connections.

B. Then the same person asked again:

Q. I think it is also true to say that a person's character depends on his associations. Therefore, if I associate with high society, should I not become high rank myself?

A. Our personality follows the shape of our associates. If you become friends with an honest person, you will become honest. But if you become friends with people of high rank, you will acquire their tendency to be very proud. Therefore, if you are a merchant with a mind of high rank, naturally you can't succeed in your business.

There might be exceptions to this during very chaotic times in society, such as war. During ordinary times, if you become lazy about your job and become friendly with people of high rank, there is no order of success. A fool who doesn't know his limitations and thinks it is his own honor to associate with honorable people is actually losing his grace. It is another story if you serve high society but remain very humble. When you pass by a stone Buddha without bowing or showing respect, you are losing His grace, so always be modest. Therefore, if you become friendly with people above you, you will lose even more grace.

#8 Physiognomy By Itself Doesn't Always Work

A. Honesty Is the Origin of Physiognomy

Q. A physiognomist told me that I would have much

happiness and wealth, but I still remain very poor and and have big difficulties. I'm wondering whether physiognomy is always right?

A. Being honest is more important than your appearance. If you are dishonest, your physiognomy is also dishonest. Your structure and features are alive and changing. If people with good physiognomy always enjoyed good fortune, there would be no point discussing it.

Even if your structure indicates good fortune, unless you are modest and refrain from bad behavior, it is no different than having poor structure. I can say that physiognomy is alive and moving like living things. This aspect of diagnosis and fortune-telling should be recognized. Even if someone has very poor features, they will enjoy happiness and wealth if they are modest. Behavior makes things change. I know a few men with good features who had to go to jail after being dishonest. Our fortune depends on how we think.

That's why I don't talk so much about fortune or misfortune when discussing physiognomy. I stress the order of heaven and earth's great, wonderful shining grace. It is most important to control your body and mind. My way of physiognomy focuses on that. People have been talking about fortune and misfortune since ancient times, but it's only for beginner's study. If someone is told that he will have good fortune, and indulges, then he will end up spoiling his grace. If someone is told that he will have misfortune lying ahead, he becomes easily discouraged and loses *ki*. This is the usual ignorance of small people. If if we forecast good fortune to a big person, he becomes happy, too. That's the nature of human emotion. Therefore, the physiognomist should not tell the person's fortunes or misfortunes.

You can go to a fortune teller if you like, but just listen to him. Ask him what is the best way to manage your job or family. Just listen to his advice of how to control yourself and your family.

Always think that your physiognomy is the worst and unluckiest, be humble and modest, and store the virtue of heaven and earth. As you accumulate virtue, your bad features will naturally change to good ones. Just concentrate on saving and storing virtue to heaven and earth.

B. The Five Virtues of the Mind[27]

Q. You talk only about health and food but never about the five cardinal virtues. If someone's health is strong and full of vitality and his food is right, but he doesn't have these five virtues, I don't think he has really mastered himself. Do you agree?

A. The five virtues are the branches. The origin of the tree of life — the roots and trunk — is to practice the order of virtues in heaven and earth. If we can make someone understand the order, then the five virtues will naturally come to him. We can say human life comes from heaven's grace and is nourished by earth's grace. Whatever sustains our life originated from heaven and earth's grace. When understanding the order of heaven and earth's grace, you naturally respect your parents' grace. You also take care of life and food, and the five virtues automatically come to you. That's why when great persons eat, their understanding of the order of nature becomes great and peaceful. But small people do not respect food, and therefore they destroy heaven's grace and attract poverty and difficulties.

C. Q. You say good and bad physiognomy changes according to the mind or heart. But don't good and bad fortune still clearly exist?

A. Life is at the same time both real and empty. That's why in my school of physiognomy, natural order itself contains neither good nor bad fortune. But if we understand the order of heaven and earth's grace and know that food is the origin, we can diagnose good or bad fortune. This is the correct way to practice diagnosis. That's why people who don't understand life don't know what the correct food for them is. If their food is correct, they will understand the order of heaven governing all phenomena. Therefore their mind becomes clear and steady, and then they can control their bodies and manage to accumulate wealth. Unless your food is correct, your life won't stabilize and you will become empty. If your food is correct, then your life and fortune will automatically become full. That's why I say humans should know the natural order of everything. It's important to understand this and practice.

Physiognomy follows this great order of heaven and earth. One who understands this order, as I have said before, will be humble and modest in his way of eating. If your eating is correct, your mind won't wander around, and you can understand more quickly the order of nature. I can say that in heaven and earth, there are five different kinds of *ki*, and a man has five virtues, and everything observes this universal order.

If your mind is floating and unsettled, you don't understand and know how to use this order, and you aren't fully developed. If you do not clearly see this order and act from it, you are losing heaven and earth's grace and your own physiognomy. Therefore, to have correct food is the most important thing. Food is the origin of nourishment for both body and mind. Unless you nourish your body properly, you can't understand the order of nature. People who are not modest in respect to food are like people living in darkness without any light.

#9 One Who Feels Sorry to Lose Just One Grain Tends to Eat One Extra Bowl of Food

A. True Hidden Virtue

Q. Ancient people have mentioned yin virtue. I'm ignorant and can't yet grasp the true meaning. Please explain about real yin virtue.

A. A man of real yin virtue would not care even if grains fell on the ground. If food is sufficient and just right for your stomach, don't worry about disgarding what is wasted. If you use anything too much, sun and moon, heaven's grace, will not forget. That is important to remember. This is called real, true yin virtue. One who does not know yin virtue feels very sad to see one grain left on the ground, but he would eat an extra bowl if it tasted good. Such persons often express sorrow to see one grain thrown away, but they don't understand how sad it is they themselves are taking an extra bowl.

What kind of merit lies in eating extra food? None. Even worse, the body suffers and yin virtue declines. Such type of people are truly ignorant of yin virtue and lose grace. They are called ignorant. It has been said that heaven doesn't create someone without wealth, but if there is life, food follows. If food ends, then life ends. That's why if you eat even one extra bowl of food, however small, you are destroying the heavenly order of grace. If you eat too much, you spoil your life's grace. Someone like this is "blind with his eyes open." His eyes do not fuction to see true wisdom. A proverb calls someone like that "a master with his eyes open who fell into a well."

B. **Q.** **Sensei, you are recommending that we refrain from eating a big quantity of food. But sometimes we are invited to dinner and are served a lot of food. If we eat that food, are we destroying our virtue?**

A. Yes, it's very bad. Being a guest with many fancy dishes set before him, he tends to eat them all because he thinks food will be wasted unless eaten. He does not know foods enter the stomach and are discharged in the feces. It's wrong just to be afraid of wasting food in front of you. A true-hearted person will throw away the food he doesn't need. This is yin virtue. If you throw away your leftover food, you may help some beings with life. Feces cannot nourish life. It may look like wasting food but it is not. Other people may not notice, but this is true yin virtue.

This is heaven and earth's virtue and grace coming down to you. Giving is virtue. The words for bestowing virtue, *toku*, and receiving, *toku*, have the same sound. Giving therefore is receiving. That's why you shouldn't eat even one mouthful of extra food if it isn't right. And you can accumulate yin virtue of heaven and earth. Even one extra mouthful ends up as stool and destroys your grace in the end. There are many who do not succeed but remain poor because they are not practicing the order of virtue.

Of course, as a general rule food shouldn't be wasted. We should use it up, even a little bit of what is left. People who are not wasteful of food accumulate a large store of heaven and earth's grace. It is called yin virtue because it is practiced unnoticed by the people around you. But later your virtue will come back as yang good news, and you will be famous.

#10 If You Don't Care for Food Well, You Can't Become a Buddha after Death.[28]

A. Features of a Person Who Dies without Being Noticed

Q. I saw a physiognomist who told me I would die by accident or by the side of the road. I worry about dying like this. Do I really have such diagnostic signs of misfortune?

A. People die such unknown deaths, or no one notices or cares about them because they wanted to. It is not owing to their physiognomic structure. Not only human beings, but also other things come to such an end, too. If you aren't humble in whatever you use and throw away things or use them carelessly, you will automatically reap the karma from such acts and end up suffering and dying yourself. This we call "dying in the field." Grasses and trees that are burnt are transformed into ashes and return to the soil. This is called "returning to Buddha." If the plants end like this, it is very good. But if you are careless and sometimes just throw the plants away because of impurity, they cannot return to the soil quickly. They will decay just like bones that are thrown away, and it will not be easy for them to return to their origin in the soil. We call such an end "death in the field." If an old tree is dirty, we should purify it with fresh water, burn it and make ashes, and return it to the soil. That is called true yin virtue. If you take care of things like this, even if your original structure has signs of death in the field, you will escape bad fortune and enjoy happy old age.

In the case of food, after proper preparation and eating, it becomes feces and is returned to the soil. This, too, we call returning to Buddha. If food is thrown out and doesn't return to the soil easily, but is allowed to ferment and rot because people waste it, it will not return to Buddha. This is a "death in the field" of food. Also allowing each food, even red leaves, to fully mature or ripen before eating is yin virtue. For human beings, the universe is creating many things with the sun's grace and the moon's grace. If you are handling things badly, you are not appreciating the sun and moon and are not following the order of nature. Such a person will suffer, especially in his old age and die. He will "die in the field."

If you understand the virtue of everything and accumulate yin virtue every day, you will become a graceful person. There were many graceful people in society; they were not born like this but accumulated grace through their strong effort. It did not happen by accident. Natural grace comes to your family. The grace of your society is manifested by your actions. A foolish person doesn't understand this order of virtue. They destroy their grace every day and blame heaven and themselves. They naturally will decline more and more, losing even the virtues accumulated for them by their ancestors.

People require three things — food, clothing, and shelter. They are like the three legs of a tripod. Like happiness, wealth, and longevity, they automatically come together. It is like having a graceful relationship with true relatives. If you have no grace and are not getting on with a relative, it's very bad to end up poor and suffering. Your relatives may look like you, but if you don't understand and take care of them, they will run away without any warning. Relatives with very simple food may be helping you now, but eventually they will say bad words at dinner to you, and they will run away. When a relative of good fortune sees this incident with regret and comes to talk to you, you attack his words. You further would change to nice clothes and go to a pleasure house to indulge with other idlers. Eventually your heart and life will be in jeopardy. An attack will come very close to you. Suddenly your former servants — food, clothing, and shelter — attack in force, and you are very ill. They march into your castle of life and attack your true nature. You end up poor and short-lived. At the end, you wear clothes made of an old flag and have to abandon your castle. You end up with a cane, walking the streets aimlessly, wasting and degrading your family name.

B. How to See Whether Someone's True Nature Is Good or Bad

Q. We say that human nature is good, but from birth babies love to drink their mother's milk. Is this bad? If humans' true nature is really good, they wouldn't want to eat food and just receive their nourishment directly from nature just like the grasses and trees. Do you call human nature good? Do you think good or bad exists in human nature?

A. As trees and grasses suck up water, a newborn baby naturally wants to eat. Suppose you pick a flower and put it in water, the flower naturally attracts the water to bloom. As we see from these examples, for everything that lives, it is natural to eat, and it is neither good nor bad. The purpose of eating is to nourish mind and body. Therefore, if you don't mind to eat simple, modest, natural foods, you are practicing good eating habits. If you indulge in rich food, we call it eating with attachment. Eating with attachment will destroy your good nature. It's bad food. There is no bad in true human nature. But by eating badly, you are destroying yourself. From bad eating habits, you end up destroying your family, mind, and body. That's why my physiognomy emphasizes a humble and modest way of eating.

#11 Secret of Physiognomy Is *Horen Ge-Kyo*[29]

Everything Has Spirit (*Myo*) and Structure (*Ho*)

Q. Sensei, you are always saying body and mind are *myo ho*, the invisible subtleness and physical order. What is *myo* and what is *ho*?

A. All phenomenon are nothing but *myo ho*, the invisible subtleness and physically appearing order. In manifestation, there are both visible existence and invisible force. The invisible one doesn't have form, but we can all clearly perceive it. We call this formlessness "subtle beauty," and it is mind. Existence has visible form. Every visible form has order. That's why we say body has order and mind has beauty. Whatever has order and form will eventually perish. This is called the Tao of Order. It also governs physiognomy. Every character originates with the mind and clearly reveals subtle beauty. Our body and mind itself reflect the beauty and order of nature as a whole. The universe is full of these. Every day, without exception, we are receiving heaven and earth's beauty and the order of society .

B. That Structure Has All *Myo Ho* (Invisible and Visible Order)

Q. In geomancy, the northeast direction between the Bull and Tiger in the zodiac is called the original direction for physiognomy. It is called the starting point. Is this true or not?

A. Geomancy and physiognomy depend on and start from a very faint balance between yin and yang. It is so faint that it is difficult to explain this subtleness — *myo*. At the end of great yin, very faint yang appears. The position of the tiger stands at the verge of the beginning of the rising sun or great yang, when the energy changes from yin to yang [between the cow and tiger in the zodiac]. We call this point beauty or mind [*myo*]. From this subtle beauty, *ki* energy is produced and circulates, forming the tiger (small yang, in the east), ending up in the cow, great yin. Here is the gate of *ki* energy — the entrance, birthplace, or capital of life and death. We call the northeast *ki-mon*, the demon gate. The words for *ki energy* and *demon* have the same pronunciation, and both are invisible forces.[30]

We can say that all geomancy and physiognomy is based on beauty and order. That's why I worship all sects of religion. Religious people study geomancy and physiognomy and understand. That's why if you are religious and study geomancy, you can understand your own religion more deeply and can lead society better. Please guide people to this deeper meaning and value of astrology and directionology. The deepest understanding of geomancy can be found in *Hokke-kyo*.[31] Please ask monks who studied this.

C. Q. Sensei, you say everything changes. Everything is born and dies. You say things without structure are born between the sheep and monkey, opposite to the tiger which is the sign of birth and death. Why do you say this?

A. The sheep is at the end of the yang phase of the sun. The

73

monkey is at the beginning of yin starting into big yin. Someone newly born receives *ki* energy from the soil of the monkey and becomes yang when encountering the horse's yang fire, then dies, and returns to the soil of the sheep. Everything is born in soil and returns to soil.

We call this back door of the northeast *ki-mon*. To our eyes, there are more trees than anything else in this world. Trees are the origin. The life and death of trees and grasses are in the sheep and monkey.

D. The tao of physiognomy lies in seeing how the person's thinking works when seeing him still and then in teaching him in the most effective way to obtain shining grace. We make him steadier from where he is already standing. Also, we make him understand the importance of standing as steady as a big flat stone. This is the essence of physiognomic study.

Physiognomy is always changing. Therefore, if you predict that someone with good structure will have good fortune, while one with bad structure will experience misfortune, this ordinary way of looking at physiognomy is dead. Real order is moving, alive, dynamic. Such is also true in physiognomy. If you don't use this moving, changing, living essence of physiognomy, you will be destroying people. In diagnosis, you should abandon your own thoughts to heaven and then diagnose the person. If you diagnose from your own energy, you will eventually be punished from heaven. Avoid always trying to change heaven's *ki* energy.

E. Disorder in your sexual relations will destroy your good fortune. If a wife has a lover, disorder will show up in her physiognomy and will spoil her future. I've seen such diagnostic signs appearing even after some years and show up on a corpse after death. Ordinarily when life is finished, the color of blood disappears, but someone with such a secret lover will retain the sign of disorder in their blood even after being buried. Such bad relationships affect your reincarnated life. From observing their structures, I can say that many men in society have such signs. And all women, without exception, have such signs. That's why I have a wife, but I don't regard her as a true wife. In Japanese, the word for woman, *fujin*, is also pronounced like the word for disorder. When a wife is good, she is like mother. When she is bad, she is like a strong demon. You should be careful.

Book III

#1 Worshipping the Sun Every Morning as a Way to Longevity

A. The Way of Living to One Hundred

People who are weak, sick, and short-lived should always honor the rising sun. After practicing this, your mind and body will become strong and you can realize long life. If you do this every day, it is very easy to reach a hundred years of longevity.[1]

By absorbing the strong energy of the morning sun, you will never fail to have *Hankon Fumetsu*. There is another way to longevity: taking the remedy of *o sei seki zui* and then honoring the rising sun.[2] These methods are the practice of a *sennin*, a free man.[3] However, it should not ordinarily be taught.

Even if you don't take the special remedy and practice *Hankon Fumetsu*, honoring the rising sun every day is the same as practicing the free man's technique. Naturally you will attain longevity. That's why I can say repeatedly, please honor the sun every day. I did not create this method myself. When I was traveling all over Japan to study, at age twenty-five, I met a stranger, a very unusual man in the east, who taught me the *sennin's* way of life to keep longevity. I show you this method out of my yin virtue.

People who are weak, sick, or short-lived should practice this way of longevity for one hundred days and learn the effectiveness of it. The method applies to both upper class and lower class. Taking care of yourself is most important. Of course, individual differences are there. Originally my features told a very short life. I would die before thirty. But I studied this way and was able to extend my life. I didn't really wish to live long myself, but honoring the sun every day, I've lived twenty years longer than I was expected to. Also I have taught this method to many people, including some who were sick, weak, and short-lived who became free from sickness and extended their life. I would really like everyone to try this way. I have also taught it to several people who have gone on to extend their life. That's why I have confidence to teach everyone.

B. From a young age, I heard that physiognomy is a *sennin's* technique. When I decided to study physiognomy at twenty-one, I naturally tried to find a *sennin* and a technique teacher. To seek such a person, I traveled all over Japan's many provinces but couldn't find any master. I hid myself in the deep mountains and meditated in many temples and pagodas. I asked the monks and priests about longevity and physiognomy, but no one could reveal the *sennin* technique. But in my twenty-fifth year, in Oshu, around Kinka-san, by chance I encountered a *sennin*.[4] I studied directly with him for one hundred days. I learned the hidden essence of physiognomy and the way of longevity. Even ordinary people who practice this way can automatically live to be a hundred very easily.

C. When an ordinary person wants to practice the *sennin* technique, he doesn't need to eat fruit, roots, and seeds like a *sennin* but may eat the five grains and animal food and sake and ordinary food, and still he can attain longevity.

D. Please study the *sennin's* book and improve your understanding.[5]

E. This book contains the *sennin's* essence. But in Japan, teaching from this book is very rare, and understanding it is rarer still. But this text includes some wonderful, unusual parts. Nevertheless, the book was written later, and there are some mistakes.

Retsu Sen Den's technique makes use of the moving energy of heaven, but if one is too greedy for this energy, he will receive punishment or a reaction from the North Star's Three Lights.[6] There is a way to avoid such misfortune. Also every person has his own way of virtue. One technique the *sennin* teaches you may be good only for you. Even if you tell the technique to other people, it will have no effect. It may even be worse for them and could be punished by the North Star's Three Lights. That's why even when I tell a special technique to someone, I am still not disclosing to him what my teacher taught me. I give only one special technique of virtue to each person. Some people have said they are my disciples and studied with me and are teaching my methods. But they are not really sincere and have no effect. I didn't make the rules but am following the *sennin* who wanted me to obey this rule strictly.

F. I can tell you when I was traveling, I changed my name five times. After hiding in the deep mountains, I taught physiognomy in villages twice, then used the name So O Zan.[7] After spending some time in shrines and in temples in the deep mountains, I experienced deep understanding. I went out to villages, then called myself Namboku Do[8] or Namboku An[9] or Nanbokuji.[10] Sometimes I became more arrogant and put the two together. After becoming a little famous, I wore a priest's robe to travel as So O Zan Nan Boku Ji. I looked very strange and people sometimes laughed at me and regarded me as a demon physiognomist. I changed my common name of Kagiya Kumataro[11] to Mizuno Syukei[12] and later Mizuno Namboku.[13] Long ago, you may have heard about me by one of these names. This is how it came about.

#2 With No Appetite, Don't Eat

Drinking a Lot of Sake and Eating Greedily Is Behaving Just like an Insect Who Loves the Fire

Q. I don't feel well. Food has no taste. But without eating, I can't nourish my mind and body. Do you find any sign of sickness in me?

A. If you don't have an appetite, don't eat. The reason you don't have an appetite is that your stomach has always been full. If you eat three times a day, then eat twice. If you normally eat twice a day, have only one meal. If you are hungry, the food, even simple, tastes good. If you observe a modest way of eating every day, your food will always taste good. If you are moderate, even without a side dish accompanying your grain, still you will keep your appetite and enjoy eating. But if you are not moderate and eat a lot, even a rich dish tastes poor and too simple. If you feel no taste, don't eat for a day. If you skip a day, then even without side dishes, but just a pinch of salt, your appetite will automatically increase. I can say that not eating to full capacity is the most wonderful way of all. If your stomach is partly empty, your *ki* energy remains healthy, and your mind works well. If you understand this but still drink and eat a lot, you are just doing bad, and you know it's bad. Everything follows this order. Unless you understand this, you are just like an insect who loves and flies into the fire.

#3 If You Are Modest about Food in This Life, You Will Be Rewarded in the Next Life

A. Cause and Effect in the Three Worlds of Past, Present, and Future

Q. I haven't had a child yet. After my death, to whom shall I leave my wealth, which has accumulated from my modest way of life with virtue. That's why I am enjoying a very luxurious way of life now. I no longer care what happens to me after I die. My virtue is to enjoy my wealth now all to myself.

A. That is very bad. Your spirit is never born and never dies. It is eternal. Once you come to this world, you will return again in human form after you die. We come back not just once, but thousands and even millions of times. The cycle repeats itself endlessly. Human beings have *inga*, or karma.[14] *In* means cause, and *ga* means effect. If you cause something bad in this life, you will reap the effect sometime. If you do something good and accumulate virtue, then that will return to you in the future. That present virtue creates your future happiness and comfort in the world. However, if you do something bad in this world and spoil your grace, you will suffer in the next world. People like you just keep their body when they are reborn but don't receive any fortune from heaven. They can't enjoy the luxurious life they left behind. They won't have a penny. That's why everything depends on what you do in the present life. If you are very modest, naturally you will become like a Bodhisattva. If you don't help yourself, who can really help you? I talk about being modest in food and drink and in all material things. If you practice these, they will be a tremendous help in the present and future. They are not my own ideas but come from Buddhist teachings. You should go to Buddhist monks and listen more deeply to what they have to say.

B. Modest Food Helps Your Descendents

Q. From a young age, I have been very modest in my way of eating. But I am still very poor and am barely able to feed my wife and child. Is there something else beyond food that is causing this?

A. There are many such fools who don't know physiognomy. I can see from your physiognomy that you didn't receive much grace from heaven but have signs of a beggar. But because from a young age you have been very modest, heaven has automatically extended its grace to you. Therefore, you don't need to beg food in this life. If someone has a physiognomy like this and eats aggressively, even a man born into a rich family would eventually lose heaven's grace and at the end of his life surely have to beg his food. Also, your original physiognomy shows you were destined to remain single and lonely.[15] But you have your own children. Later in life a child will help you obtain food. Even if you are very wealthy, unless you have a child or grandchild, your old age will be very poor. You have been very modest from a young age, so when you grow old, you can depend on your child and won't need to beg food. Don't worry about not being so rich. Just understand what is enough for you and become more and more modest about your food. Then you can receive more of heaven's grace and leave it to your descendents' success. I can assure you that whatever grace you accumulate is for you as well as your descendents. It doesn't belong to anyone else.

#4 The Size of Your Plate or Bowl Depends on Whether You Are Big or Small

Q. I do not use my body so much for physical work, but I'm an aggressive, big eater. I can't control my food. From today I have decided to eat only two large bowls a day. If I do this for three years, can I become rich and enjoy a long life?

A. Whether one is rich or poor and lives in the busy city or countryside, the size of the bowl depends on his limitations. City people tend not to do as much physical work, so usually a small bowl is to be used when eating. Mountain and country people are more physically active, and their bowls are much bigger. You will notice that noble persons use valuable plates or bowls, while laborers don't use small ones. The size of dishes is governed by heaven's order according to the individual. From olden days we called valuable plates or bowls *tenmoku*.[16] It is best if your dishes match your limitations. The five grains are the origin and foundation of the human diet. The five grains are associated with the five energies. We call this *go ki*, which also means five dishes or bowls.[17] I mentioned already that a limited amount of food is given to you from heaven. If we observe these limitations, we nourish our heaven-sent life. Heaven sees one and decides the quantity of his food. That's why we traditionally call dishes or bowls *tenmoku*. *Ten* means heaven, while *moku* means eye.

B. The Theory of Eating Only to Eighty Percent Capacity

Q. I heard that if we are modest we will eat to only eighty percent of our stomach's capacity. How can one tell if it is eighty percent full?

A. Big or small, strong or weak, everyone's body has different limitations and requirements. Someone will be satisfied with only two or three bowls. Someone else will need four or five bowls to become full. If your *hara* is satisfied after eating three bowls, you should eat only two and one half. That is eighty percent. It's very good to be strict in your food. If you eat 100 percent, that brings you misfortune. Just eating to eighty percent is best. They say: "Normally if you really like to eat, the gate of your stomach, spleen, and pancreas will open and you can receive food." If you eat to only eighty percent, say two to two and one half bowls, that is good for your *hara*. Then immediately those organs will shut. We call this heaven's natural order. But if you fill your stomach and other organs 100 percent, the gate of the pancreas cannot close. With eighty percent food, it can close nicely. An immodest person eats afer the gate is closed, and the food has to stay before actually digesting in the organs and stagnates. This is the origin of sickness and misfortune. With this view, the cause of people becoming sick and experiencing misfortune is always from food and drink. That is the basic cause. Even a great or wise person becomes sick or misfortunate because of not really being modest. If you are modest, you won't experience these. If you are not modest, we can't say you are truly great or wise. Such people could be called demons. If you are very modest, you will not get sick except for catching a cold of bad energy sometimes.

C. Origin of Peace and Happiness in Past, Present, and Future

Q. Sensei, you say the secret of life in the three worlds of past, present, and future is in modest food. But Nanki Moku Jiki Shonin says he is going to release his bad karma and improve his future destiny by meditating and chanting.[18] Is he correct? I don't think modesty in food is the only way to attain peace and happiness in the three worlds.

A. Chanting is endlessly precious. People don't know there are many Buddhist monks living in rich temples, wearing fancy red robes, carrying elaborate beads, and just chanting without thinking. Nanki Moku Jiki is not like this. He has no house or temple and wears only very simple, poor clothing, and he walks around from village to village. Ordinary people love and worship him. Which approach is better? Maybe Nanki Moku Jiki looks foolish, but he doesn't eat very much himself and extends his grace to heaven and earth. That's why ordinary people automatically worship him. There is no other reason. Everything he accomplished he did for himself by accumulating virtue from his food. A Buddhist who can't control himself but eats to his full capacity every day and uses up his grace from heaven and earth loses his grace from heaven in the end. He will not be looked up to by people as Moku Jiki Shonin. I conclude there is nothing more important than food.

Among the Jodo Shin Shu sect, chanting *"Namu Amida Butsu"* is excellent and the essence of their teaching.[19] These six sounds are perfect and true. *Na* makes the sound of long "ah" and *mu* makes "u." "Ah" comes again with "ah" in *mi* and "da" into *a*. In *Butsu*, there is "u" and "u." The chanting satisfies the basic vowels. Jodo Shin Shu monks are permitted to marry and eat animal food. But if someone follows this, he destroys his grace. No one in other sects or other people actually practices food modesty like Moku Juki Shonin. To observe modesty is the essence of his teachings. It is the central practice. We can say that if you are modest and humble in your way of eating in the present world and extend your grace from heaven and earth, you can release bad karma from your past life. As a result you can extend your present life and enjoy good fortune, too. Because of modesty in this life, you will be able to attain peace and happiness in the next life. And at the end of your present life, you will automatically die peacefully. They say: "Our mind at the end of our present life creates our next life." If someone doesn't suffer at the end of his life, his next life will be happy and peaceful. Anyone who is modest in his eating now, extending his virtue to heaven and earth, can benefit in his next life. In Buddhist teachings, there are rules about decreasing the amount of food you eat. Those rules in the present life are to improve the next life. I can say that life in the present world and the future world depend on nothing but a modest and humble way of eating. These are not just my words. They are written in the sutras.

#5 Buddhist Teachings for Improving Yourself by Observing a Moderate Way of Eating

"Namu Amida Butsu" and Food

Q. You have said that even if we chant *"Namu Amida Butsu"* day and night but don't eat modestly, we aren't following the Buddha's teachings. I have listened to many Buddhist masters, but none of them has talked about this. Are you are not misrepresenting Buddha's true way?

A. Buddha's teachings are yin. Their purpose is to control our *ki* energy. That's why the starting point is in moderate food. A disturbed mind is caused by the way we eat. If you are modest about food, your mind will be quiet and peaceful. If the mind is quiet and stabilized, it's easy to attain tao. But if you eat much sake and animal food, your consciousness becomes too aggressive and you do something not good. If you eat too much, your mind is naturally stagnated, and your *ki* energy becomes heavy, and your mind wanders, and you can't attain tao. In their study and practice, Buddhist monks cut down their food by not eating after 6 p.m. This is nothing but making their *ki* energy quiet and controlling their mind. Even day and night you chant *"Namu Amida Butsu,"* if your mind remains floating and wandering, you cannot attain Buddha's heart. If you are modest, cut down one bowl of food from your usual three bowls and give it to Buddha, and then if you chant, your mind will become very peaceful and stable. Then your stable mind makes you attain tao very easily. But if you overeat, chant, and pray for the future, without offering any food to Buddha, that is very bad. It is not necessary to set aside one bowl of food for Buddha. Just reduce what you eat and save it for the future. That satisfies Buddha's heart. I can say that observing a modest way of eating and saving food for the present and future are the essence of Buddha's teachings. You'd better read the *Riku Go kyo Sutra*. The sutra does tell you this.

B. A Lot of Sake Makes Life Short and Sick

Q. I am able to moderate my eating, but I really love sake. I can't moderate that. Should sake be harmful to my health? [20]

A. If you drink a little bit of sake, your *ki* will increase and your circulation will improve. But if you drink much, definitely you will shorten your life. God doesn't like you to drink a lot of sake. When people have a party, in the beginning they drink a little bit. At that time its taste is good and everyone smiles and is relaxed. But later when they drink too much, people experience a bitter taste and they suffer. This is the greedy way of drinking and the way leading to suffering for both body and mind. God suffers and automatically you frown from drinking too much. Intuitively you are also afraid of heaven then. You hit your head and breathe out "ah." Shouldn't a lot of sake be disliked by God? When ordinary people get drunk, the next day they always have trouble with their stomach. At this time you understand that too much sake is not good for your health. But then you take medicine to cure this imbalance. Your suffering goes away and you forget, and again you do the same thing. After you do like this for several years, even blessed with physiognomic signs of longevity, you tend to shorten your life and become sick. Please be careful and modest with sake.

#6 Poor People Should Not Practice Rich People's Hobbies

A. To Have a Caged Animal or Not?

Q. You have taught if one has physiognomic signs of longevity and wealth in later life, but still is poor himself and enjoys keeping a nightingale in a cage at home, he will not succeed in society. Also such a person will face difficulties later in life. But Buddha's teaching is not to kill living things. How would he not become prosperous?

A. Keeping a bird is the enjoyment of upper class people, someone very rich who doesn't need to make a living. If you are still poor and low class and have the same pleasures of upper class society, you will spoil nature's grace. That's why even if you have such a good physiognomy, your life will not be successful. If you don't have any further ambition than keeping a bird, then you will never succeed in any direction.

A successful man made himself successful because he enjoyed it. He has controlled himself and his house and contributed to society.

Toward that end, he is happy to prolong the family name that he inherited from the ancestors. This type of person doesn't really enjoy keeping a bird or indulging in other idle pleasures. If you have not yet made your way in life but are enjoying the pleasures of upper class hobbies, you are seeking out poverty for yourself. You will create misery and failure for yourself. If you are enjoying the bird just a little bit, it will eventually interfere with your life and work. Many things will not go smoothly. One who doesn't put his mind into his job tends to look elsewhere for pleasure.

Unless you control yourself, like the bird, you will die without realizing your dream. If you seek enjoyment, then the rest of your life automatically will suffer. If you do not seek enjoyment, you will not experience suffering later in life. Therefore, don't seek only enjoyment. Put your whole effort into your work and enjoy. Then you will succeed and climb up.

#7 Working at Night Is Very Unfortunate and Getting Up Late Makes for Poverty and a Short Life

A. Q. You have taught that even with bad physiognomy, if one gets up early in the morning, his fortune will gradually become better. But I'm a craftsman and usually work till late at night. I can't get up so early.

A. Working late at night is very bad. You'd better go to sleep at 8 p.m. If you wish to work four hours later at night, instead get up four hours earlier the next morning. Go to sleep at 8 p.m., then get up four hours early and work with a light on as at night. This way you use the sun's rising energy. When you go together with the rising sun, automatically the movement of your own *ki* will become better. Gradually you will become rich and enjoy a long life. That is the order of nature.

Even if you work four hours at night, getting up late four hours does not make you feel good, and you can't handle anything well. When you wake up four hours early, the atmosphere is very quiet. Your mind and body feel much stronger, and you don't feel sleepy. In this way you can do your job better and more efficiently. Isn't it because the sun's early morning energy is very good? Sleeping late in the morning is the origin of poverty and short life. You must be very, very careful.

B. Q. You have taught that even if someone's physiognomy indicates a short life, he can extend his life by receiving small growing yang *ki*. How can I receive such successful *ki*?

A. Controlling my way of eating, I have now become fifty, and people say I look younger than my age, and my bone structure shows signs of longevity. I do not know what will happen tomorrow, but I have already extended my life by twenty years. I encourage everyone to be modest about food and sexual activity and to honor their parents.

#8 When Woman Recognizes Signs of Her Good Fortune, It Changes to Misfortune

Q. Sensei, you have said that women shouldn't discuss physiognomy. But the Emperor, the Shogun, and other lords have wives and mistresses. Why are they not able to discuss physiognomy?

A. Man and woman are yang and yin. Therefore both show signs of physiognomy.[21] Because Japan is a country of peace and harmony, ladies hold the power. But yin has to always follow yang. That's why by following the lead of man and supporting him, woman can grow. There are many such women in the upper class, but few in the lower class. These women should not discuss physiognomy. Upper class women would not naturally discuss it. Only lower class women want to discuss it.

If we tell an ordinary woman that she will have good fortune, she becomes too proud. Her arrogance eventually disturbs her husband. The house is no longer peaceful and the family suffers. She thinks from that time her physiognomy is very good and her husband's is very bad and that's why they are suffering. She blames her husband. This is always the way ordinary women think. Even with a husband with bad physiognomy, if the wife is modest and humble, she will automatically help him succeed. Such is the marvelous order of heaven and earth.

In my way of physiognomy, I didn't tell an ordinary woman she has good fortune. I show her instead the order of nature. Also noble and upper class women have very nice manners and follow their husbands. Her good or bad fortune always shows up in her husband. As it has been said: "A country's disorder is not created by heaven but by women." That's why whether from high or low class, women have to be very careful and modest.

#9 Even Though You Are Very Humble and Modest, Heaven May Still Test You

A. Buddha's Virtue of Grace

Q. I heard that when Buddha was training on the snow mountain, he ate only six grains of millet a day. Can only six grains nourish his stomach?

A. Nothing that lives can survive without eating. Even Sakya-muni Buddha could live with only six grains of millet. But in the snow mountains he cut down his food and gave this to worship heaven and earth. In this way, he prayed and realized his wishes. By offering his food to heaven, his great virtue created enough grace to fill up the entire world. His prayers and wishes were granted at the same time. Since then his teachings have continued to expand. We don't need to think that he lived on only six grains of millet. But we can understand that he was very humble and modest about food. To show the limit of what food shall be, he is said to have taken only six grains as a symbol. In any case, for ourselves, we should cut down our quantity of food and offer the rest to heaven and earth. This is the biggest hidden virtue. The essence of Buddha's teachings is based on extending our yin virtue by controlling our food. Keeping food consumption under control is his number one practice. If you really wish to be humble in your way of eating, Buddha's teachings are excellent. If you wish to realize your wishes and dreams, please be modest and cut down the amount of food you eat and give the food you saved to the North Star and pray for whatever tao you wish to do. Then heaven will naturally grant your prayers and wishes.

B. Heaven's Test

Q. Because of wanting to be famous, I'm keeping very modest and humble. But my fortune is growing worse and worse. I'm suffering now. It looks like fortune or misfortune does not actually depend on humility. If we really have strong destiny, should we not be successful regardless?

A. Even when someone is successful in his own tao while being very strict and modest, heaven sometimes gives him more and more difficulties. That will enable him to find another tao in life. Great men do not regard this as a difficulty but keep going. That's why they end up being famous in the world. But a small man can't handle these heaven-sent difficulties and, with his mind disordered, blames heaven. That's why he attracts more and more troubles and ends up not succeeding and vanishing away, especially if he is very modest in his way of life but not modest in his way of eating. However, a small person who is modest about his food and keeps humble will not be disturbed in his mind. Modesty in food is the essence. Be very strict and modest in your way of eating and do good things, and just wait for heaven's fortune to come. Everything good or bad will come according to what you have done.

That's why *un* means "moving" or "circling." Fortune and misfortune are all returning back in a circle, whatever you are doing. That's why *un* is also returning grace. If one time you do a good deed, that good deed will return to you. Fortune and misfortune are like this, endlessly circling and coming back. That is heaven and earth's order. That's why your fortune is determined by whatever you do and follows your own actions. If you are enjoying things only for yourself, immediately suffering comes back to you. *Un* also has the meaning of working and carrying one. Even if what you have done is only faintly good, if you carry on this good deed, your virtue will eventually fill up heaven and earth. That's why someone of good deeds will never be poor or suffer.

#10 Too Luxurious Clothing and Housing Makes for Misfortune

Q. Human beings need clothing, food, and housing. If we are really modest about our food, but our clothing and house are extravagant, is our grace destroyed or not?

A. To be good, clothing and housing should depend on our social position and character. If you have extravagant clothes on, you are decorating just your outside and you will definitely suffer inside. If you are modest and respecting your limits, grace automatically comes inside. At that time, to others it may look like you are having difficulties. But inside yourself everything is going smoothly. That's why if your energy goes outward into clothing and household, your grace will definitely be less inside yourself. Someone who is very extravagant appears to be free. But if you are frugal and keep your virtue hidden on the inside, that is real wealth. If someone has true virtue inside, it doesn't show up outwardly. A person of virtue does not show this virtue outwardly. Someone who eats and drinks chaotically and is not modest about his life becomes decorative outwardly and fools ordinary people and society. Someone whose food and drink is modest knows his own limitations and will not be extravagant. Among clothing, food, and housing, food is the most important. Food's position is inside and yin. Food, therefore, should be quiet and not gourmet. Rich and luxurious food give you misfortune. Clothing and housing are outward — yang. Keeping beautiful and comfortable is good, but making them too extravagant leads to misfortune.

#11 One's Fortune Has a Lot to Do with the Sun's Movement

A. The Real Meaning of Heaven's Grace

Q. My fortune has not been good from a young age. I always have difficulties. Please tell me, on the basis of your physiognomy, whether I have heavenly grace or not.

A. Not only you but many people in the world sigh that they aren't destined for good fortune. Or sometimes they experience misfortune and complain to heaven. I can tell you, no one is without good fortune. Having a bad destiny doesn't exist because our bodies are born by heaven's yang fire. The sun's fire is circulating in our body day and night without stop. This we call *un*. *Un* is moving, circling. Fortune means life itself. That's why we say *un*, destiny, is life. We say *un mei* is fortune-life.[22] Everyone rich or poor is sharing in heaven's fortune and can live. That's why when heaven's grace ends, your life also ends. The word for life is *hito*.[23] Another meaning of *hito* is heaven's fire — the energy of the sun that is staying inside of us. Staying inside we call *to do maru*.[24] The sun (fire, *hi*) is staying inside of us.

What we call death is the fire going out. *Hi* is receding. Yang fire goes back to heaven. The word for death is *hi i*, to leave.[25] The fire has gone. As long as a person has a fire (*hi*) in himself, he is not dead (*hi i*). That's also why if someone is still alive, we can never say they have no fortune. Bettering our fortune is nothing but following the order of heaven. The sun rises in the east at the time of the position of the tiger without ever resting and is constantly cycling. Human beings should be just like the sun. If you wake up 6 a.m. and do your job like the sun, then automatically you will be moving with heaven's order, and your fortune will gradually get better. I can say the character *un* is used in *un-ten*, *un-sen*, and *un-do*, and we can say that *un* also means constant movement and turning and cycling and circulating like nature itself.[26] If you don't move on your own accord, automatically you lose your *un*, fortune. Working with your *ki* in your day-to-day job or work creates fortune. We have another expression, *un sei*.[27] *Sei* means "strongly moving." *Un sei* signifies opening the gate of fortune.

#12 Why Does Getting Up Early Improve Your Destiny?

A. Sleeping Late Harms Your Grace

Q. You have said: "If you wake up early, you will be healthy and prosperous." There must be a limited amount of life and fortune from heaven we can receive. Therefore should it not matter whether we get up early or late? Would our life and fortune not become strong or change?

A. The rising sun is small yang and has auspicious *ki* energy for progress. When people getting up receive this rising energy they automatically become healthier in both body and mind, which makes their fortune naturally prosperous. One's fortune is moving together with his *ki*. That why we call *un-ki*, the power of life, or *un-mei*, fortune.[28] If fortune is healthy, then automatically success and prosperity follow. Your healthy *ki* energy is the key and makes your fortune healthy. Therefore, someone who gets up late after the rising *ki* of the sun, even with good physiognomy, his fortune cannot be complete and he will not prosper and succeed. If in doubt, please watch someone who gets up late. They are not physically healthy, and their face color is bad. Because they are waking up later than the rising small yang *ki* of the sun, the fire they receive from heaven cannot augment their inner fire. That's why their *ki* energy is weak and their body and mind are not healthy and their face color is bad. Such a person's fortune is incomplete, and he can't climb up and advance in society.

People who get up late generally sleep about 70 percent of their life, eat and drink ten percent, and travel and enjoy themselves 10 percent. Only the other ten percent of the time is spent on the job. They may work hard day and night, but they will never prosper. Late risers tend to say up late at night and are thieves of yin and yang. Why? Because yang wakefulness changes to yin sleeping. Not only that, but sleeping in the day and playing around at night is not going with the order of nature, and their *un mei* is never fulfilled. Already the sun is rising at the time of the tiger, but still they are sleeping like a child for no use. When you wake up at 10 a.m. to do your job, you cannot do it properly because already four hours have passed from the usual time to get up. Your hands can't handle things well. The whole day's energy is stagnated as a result. If you end up doing only half a day's work, there cannot be any order, and your fortune can't improve. If you would really like to attain good fortune, whether you are high rank or low, there is no other way but getting up early, working hard, and being modest in your way of eating. If you go against these, your fortune will not be successful, and your family will soon decline. There are many such clear examples around you.

#13 Frugality Makes for Fortune, Stinginess for Misfortune

Q. I'm very frugal and that's why people feel bad about me. I have difficulty keeping employees and servants. Should I stop being frugal? Please give me your advice.

A. I think your frugality is based on stinginess. Therefore misfortune arises. A really frugal person is always careful to remember what is important and what is not important in things from one end to the other. But small people think frugality means cutting their employees' or servants' food and drink or not contributing money to charities or society. This is not frugality but stinginess. That's why people who work for you steal money and eat out. If employees talk back, it is because their master is not human. He is mixing up frugality and stinginess.

From now on you shouldn't think about frugality but heaven and earth's grace, and then don't waste anything you use. You yourself, cut down the amount of food you eat by ten percent, but don't restrict your employees. Make these as your center, and be strict. Work hard and keep watch over the household. A master of the house understands and talks to his employees and family about the importance of heaven and earth's grace. Keep the ten percent rule strictly yourself, and others in the house will notice. And the whole household will become happy and harmonious and eventually everyone will become truly frugal, and society will regard you as a wise man.

#14 If Your Food Is Modest, Then *Ki* Energy Will Open and Your Fortune Will Open

A. Master of the Mind

Q. You have said that even with diagnostic signs of a short life, if we are modest in our food, we can change that and live a long life. But from a young age, I have been greedy for food. But if that order is clear and strong, I can control myself. Please explain to me, what is the real truth and order of physiognomy.

A. Firstly, our body is just like a house. The mind is the master of the body's house. Even if you received a healthy body house from your father and mother, you can damage your health. You can become sick from an unhealthy way of life and end up destroying your body house because of your poor mind, the master of your body house. That's like an immodest master of the family ruining his ancestors' honor. If you don't take care of your body house, you will die early. If the master of a house is modest, then he can keep up the family's honor for a long time.

But even if the house is healthy, still sometimes it can face difficulties. At that time, unless the master controls himself very well, he cannot manage to make the house right. At such times of decay, the roof is damaged and the rain and sunshine get into the house. Then you cannot protect yourself from hot and cold, wind and rain. Naturally you cannot stay in the house and in the end must leave. This all comes from lack of modesty.

If you cannot control yourself and be modest, you create sickness and damage your body. Then your mind or spirit can't stay in your body and in the end must go back to heaven. Even if you are very sad about this, you cannot return again. Sometimes a doctor may fix you up, but in case of big damage even the doctor can't cure it. This all comes about because of poor mind or spirit that likes rich food and makes you an aggressive eater. You will become sick and have a short life.

You should be very fearful of heaven's order. If you are modest and control your body, your spirit, the master of the house, won't have to return to heaven. If you know this order and still eat aggressively, you are making your body house an enemy. You are spoiling yourself as if you are breaking walls, crushing the house, and pulling out the foundation. Generally, ordinary people know chaotic eating is not good for the health of their bodies, but still they drink sake endlessly and they get drunk and forget their limit. As a human being, if you don't know yourself, we say that you are ignorant. You are just like an insect flying into the fire. Such persons are no use to the world. We call someone like this *goku-tsubushi*. The meaning is "pressed, thrown away grain."

Q. You have said that if we are moderate in our food, our face color will get better and our fortune will automatically improve. I agree that food is nourishing mind and body, but I don't think it correlates with fortune.

A. Food is the foundation for nourishing mind and body. That's why if you are humble and eating modestly, the five transformation organs will become healthy, and your *hara* will automatically become better.[29] When mind and body are healthy, *ki* energy will automatically open. When the *ki* is opening, the gate of fortune will open. That's why fortune follows *ki*. That's why we say together *un ki*.[30] If you eat excessively, then your *hara* becomes bad and your *ki* becomes stagnated. If your energy is stagnated, your face color stagnates. That's why blood color automatically worsens. If good blood color is absent, the gate of fortune can't open. That's why we can say if you are really modest and humble in your way of eating, your blood color becomes better, and your fortune automatically opens. Anyway, for three years try to be modest and humble for food. If then the gate of *un ki* doesn't open, there is no order in heaven and earth, the gods don't exist, and bells and drums cannot make sound. You can also say Mizuno Namboku is an enemy of society.

#15 Wise Man without Learning, Unwise Man with Learning

A. Small Person's Training

Q. You teach that we can control ourselves and house by studying phenomena and natural order. But how can ordinary people be able to improve themselves without wise men's teachings of tao?

A. Phenomena correlate with natural order and principles. It is important to see beginning and end, center and periphery. Frugality and moderation are the starting point. If someone studies and can practice, automatically he will understand the importance of his job and house and become frugal. When small people control and take care of themselves and are not luxurious or extravagant, they will be able to manage themselves and their houses in a straight and orderly way. That is the beginning of the way of human beings to be straight and orderly. Because originally human nature is good, without learning, their mind is right. That's why there are many people who without learning old masters still respect their parents and take care of themselves. On the other hand, there are also many who have learned but don't respect their parents and cannot control themselves and just float around and die. Even very knowledgeable people who are not modest and frugal and don't work hard can't control their houses. That's why ordinary people only study daily business transactions and other job-related matters at other times. If you do that, you can control your home and master the five energies.[31] For small people, too much study is the same as not enough. Sometimes they can study too much and destroy their home. This is worse than not learning.

#16 Why a Good Person's Life Is Short and a Bad Person's Life is Long

Q. A person of deep love and care often dies early. An aggressive, bad guy, however, often enjoys a long life. Does evil extend and destroy the good for this to happen? Is this so?

A. This is all caused by the *ki* of the mind or heart.[32] The person with weak *ki* of mind has a short life. The person with strong *ki* of mind creates a long life. The person with weak *ki* of mind has no endurance and cannot compete long. Also a person of endurance cannot work at bad things for long. That's why it looks as though a good person's life is short. But we cannot always say he is really a good person. Their weak *ki* of mind made them die young. A person with strong *ki* of mind has good endurance and when he meets someone, he naturally is strong. When in occasional conflicts with other people, his energy is strong, he is able to complete things and survive. That's why a person who is called bad lives long because his *ki* of mind is strong. A truly good person reflects on himself every day and is humble, respects his elders, takes care of younger people, and doesn't dislike difficult people. Such a person is really a man of sincerity. Rarely do we see someone like that, except the emperor or a saint.

A. Secret of Longevity

Q. **I would like to extend my life and achieve longevity. What is most important?**

A. Life is given by heaven, and it is the real origin or root of mind and body. It's easy to extend life. You just have to nourish your *ki* of personality. The source of this nourishment is, of course, food. But besides food, the eyes, ears, nose, tongue, body and thinking all together must be quiet and silent. Even a very short time, being quiet and silent extends your life.

If you nourish the *ki* of your personality in this way, even for one minute, your life will be extended greatly. One who understands heaven and earth's grace will not waste anything and knows his action brings in happiness and longevity according to the order of heaven. Therefore he even enjoys more being humble and frugal, and then his mind will become peaceful, and automatically the *ki* of his personality will be nourished. He will naturally create great *ki* energy. But someone who loves sake, meat, and rich food will spoil their mind and body, and automatically he will destroy such great *ki* energy, and his life will be short. One who keeps frugal and modest, even if he was born with physiognomic signs of poverty and a short life, can extend his grace, his longevity, and his fortune according to heaven's order.

B. A Person Who Cannot Be Kept in Employment

Q. **I have not done bad things from a young age. I have only helped people. Still no one likes to hire me or keep me on a job. Why is this?**

A. Because you are not modest, people do not use you. You are just throwing yourself away. The reason for this is that because you want a lot of things without good reasons and also you waste them. Therefore nature gives retribution, and people throw you away. Not only are you thrown away by people, but if you are not modest everything will also abandon you because man and everything belong to One, in which the same order of heaven applies. When you are employed and the master does not treat you well and throws you out like dust, you hate the master. You then are a small person. When you are modest and think that you are unwise and work very hard with all your efforts for your master, even emphemerally, helping anything which may decline one day is better than *Ho Sho*.[33] In this way you can extend your happiness and life, and people will not throw you out. We can't really predict fortune or misfortune by looking only at physiognomy. Everything depends on your own humbleness and modesty.

C. **Q.** An old proverb says, "If the method of cutting food isn't right, we shouldn't eat." [34] If your teacher prepares such things which make you sick in the stomach, are you going against the tao by respecting your teacher? Is this good or bad?

A. Yes, it's really bad. Even if cutting of the food is good, and you eat too much, digestive sickness will come and disturb your tao and respect for your teacher. And even if the food is not cut correctly and you eat a small quantity, that food will help nourish your spirit and body. Your virtue then works just like medicine. But myself, I do not want to destroy heaven and earth's grace, so I eat very humble, simple food. If it's not really cut correctly, then I purify and eat it. You can see miso, tamari, sake, vinegar, and foods like that which are fermented and purified and taste good. Even after fermentation, we eat them as purified. Then they don't cause digestive problems. Also if you understand heaven and earth's grace and don't overeat, even poor food tastes good. If you appreciate its wonderful natural taste, simple food will nourish you and is better than medicine.

#17 How to Grow a Very Smart and Active Child

A. Limiting Eating and Clothing

Q. They say: "When you take care of children, don't give them dirty clothes and food that is chaotic." If we bring up children by such a rule, they will grow up and automatically become bright and smart. On the other hand, if we give them food that is not right, they will not grow up correctly or become very intelligent. That way was taught. Is it right or not?

A. In the old days, they were eating very simple food and drinking water and experiencing deep joy inside. This is certainly true. Intelligence comes from God's brightness. Intelligence doesn't depend on wearing beautiful clothing or eating rich food. Wearing fancy clothes and eating rich food doesn't let God's brightness shine to make a genius. It's high society's practice not to wear dirty clothing nor to eat food which has not been cut correctly. If you are from a lower class and copy those rules or customs of the upper class, it's against the order of heaven, and you destroy your housing even with enough food and clothing. That's why food and clothing rules depend on your social rank. You can still show intelligent *ki* even if you wear poor clothing and eat simple food. If your father and mother are very poor and their life has been too busy with day to day concerns, you may become foolish. There are some people born into poor families who become very smart and successful. The other way, there are some persons, even generals and the shogun, who were born into nobility or the upper class but are very foolish. A jewel remains a precious jewel, even when it grows in the mind. When the time comes, it will be recognized by society. Success depends on what you do.

#18 Life Has No Birth, No Death, No Beginning and No End

Ki of Mind Resides in the *Tanden*[35]

Q. Sensei, you say that even if you are born with a short life, you are free to achieve longevity. But only God decides your life. How are we able to lengthen it?

A. Life has no beginning and no end. and therefore there is no long life nor short life. As I explained before, man lives by receiving heaven's yang fire. We call this fire of the heart or spirit. While this fire of the spirit doesn't return to heaven, we shall never die. If you are moderate and take care of yourself, the fire stays well in your *tanden* and can live long. If one is not modest, the fire of the spirit cannot stay in the *tanden*. Please master knowing how not to let the fire of spirit return to heaven. Then even if your physiognomy shows a short life, you won't die early.

In the free man's text, the *sennin* is said to breath out from the ankles. The *sennin* is empty and always full with *ki* of mind in his *tanden*. The top of your foot correlates with the *san ko* on the back.[36] The *san shin* on the ankle corresponds with a point in the *tanden*.[37] If *ki* of mind stays in the *tanden* and is quiet, he can breath out from the ankles.

When you have an accident, if the *ki* of mind remains in the *tanden*, then you don't lose "fire of mind."[38] Such persons never faint. People whose fire spirit doesn't stay in the *tanden*, when they suddenly fall down from a high place exclaim, "ah." The breathing of "ah" sends their fire of the spirit back to heaven. Even if they call it, it doesn't come back. This happens because they are not modest nor humble and the spirit does not stay in their *tanden*. That's why they may have an accident and uexpected death. A man who is humble and modest has his fire of the spirit in the *tanden*. Even if he falls down from a high place, he will stop breathing as "um." His *tanden* becomes like a big rock. Then the *ki* of his spirit stays with him. Because his *ki* of the spirit wouldn't move, he doesn't faint. Therefore the fire of the spirit cannot return to heaven. We call keeping the *ki* of the spirit in the *tanden* a free man's longevity. The key to keep happiness, fortune, and longevity is in the *tanden*. Whether the *ki* of the spirit stays in your *tanden* or not depends completely on the modesty of your food.

#19 The Grace of Salt That Holds Together the Human Body

If You Waste Salt, Your Life Will Be Poor and Short

Q. Besides the five grains, what foods can we say are next important? Which are best?

A. The grace of all food is truly more than we can measure. But besides the five grains, we can say that the next important food is salt. Salt is the essence of the world. It not only exists in the ocean, but it is found all over the land. Acccording to the *ki* movement between yin and yang, it is distributed everywhere. The grace of salt makes everything hold together. Also we can say that the five grains and all other foods possess one of the five tastes. That all comes from yang salt's grace. Salt is the center or origin of the five tastes. Salt makes our bodies form and hold together. Its grace is as important as that of the five grains. Therefore, if you are carelessly handling salt or waste it, even if your physiognomy is good, your life will always be poor and short. Even someone with good fortune, if he abuses salt, will always get sick, and his life will be short. The reason, according to the order of heaven and earth, is that he is destroying the heaven-sent substance that makes the body hold together. Of course, divinity is in all phenomena. But the most gracious deities are in salt and grains. That's why I can say in Oshu, there is a shrine of the Shining God of Salt Making Pot.[39] This is a very famous metaphysical experience. If someone behaves badly at this shrine, he immediately receives punishment. Abusing salt is just like disobeying God. Be careful.

Book IV

#1 Confucian Scholars Are Not Necessarily Men of Virtue

Q. We call Sorai Ogyu and Syundai Dazai men of virtue, but people don't call them as such.[1] Are Confucian scholars not men of virtue?

A. Sorai and Dazai were not men of virtue. With their strong *ki* of mind they could study and memorize better than anyone else. That's why we call them "strong people." But no one calls these Confucian scholars men of great virtue. We say they are just strong and great, and from olden days till today we really think their *ki* of mind was higher and stronger than millions of people. There have been only a few great Confucian scholars. Small men thus cannot become strong people.

But to be a man of virtue is easy. A real man of virtue does not necessarily talk about scholarly things. In daily life, they study all phenomena around them as their book and find the order of nature. When a person really understands the order around him, he understands the importance of nature's grace. Automatically he becomes very humble and modest and naturally accumulates heaven and earth's grace. We call such a person a man of virtue. Even if such a person is very poor, his life will be rich, happy, and peaceful. Ordinary people automatically admire his virtue and follow him. After awhile, he ends up becoming famous and is called a man of virtue in the world.

That's why I can say even if a person is small and not intelligent, it's easy for him to become a man of virtue in the world if he accumulates heaven and earth's grace day to day. In this society big, strong persons are very rare. But there are many men of virtue. In studying any type of tao, except for a few strong, big persons with natural ability, becoming famous starts with accumulating heaven and earth's grace day to day.

All teachers should practice virtue. Unless you practice it, there is no way you can attain the order of nature. Without practice, you would not understand that everything originates from heaven and earth's grace, and you would just seek money and wealth. Such people don't mind to waste things and indulge in drinking sake, eating meat, and in sex. Their liver *ki* is too strong and aggressive to listen to anyone else's opinion. Sometimes they talk as though they are very knowledgable to surprise people who often approach them. Then such talkative people become very snobbish and as a result greatly disturb their own grace. Then eventually their grace is worn out, and at the end of their lives they are not ashamed to wear untidy clothes. They think themselves a great master, but ordinary people treat them like men of disturbed mind. People never follow someone who doesn't understand heaven and earth's grace. You have to be very careful. If you really wish to prosper, be disciplined and extend your grace to heaven and earth. Everything follows the order of heaven. Therefore, understand the grace of heaven and earth.

#2 Everything Is Divinely Created including Heaven and Earth

Frugality Is the Way to Tao

Q. It is said that after heaven and earth were created the deity Kuni-Toko-Tachi-No-Mikoto was born.[2] But did everything exist before him or not?

A. We sometimes talk about Kuni-Toko-Tachi-No-Mikoto, but he doesn't have a body and structure. We call the holiness of everything's virtue Kuni-Tachi-No-Mikoto. Everything comes from heaven's shining grace. From ancient times till today, this order has not changed. After the creation of heaven and earth, the first deity was born, but without phenomena his life couldn't really be nourished. That's why every phenomenon is the origin and is Kuni-Toko-Tachi-

No-Mikoto. This deity's grace is limitless. Therefore, persons who understand the grace of every phenomenon can master the order of nature and automatically worship all of creation. And they don't waste anything and are frugal. Therefore, they will receive the deity's grace at last. They will become almost one with the tao itself. That's why physiognomists should at first understand this order and carefully cultivate heaven and earth's grace day to day and work to influence society and guide people's way of life through their teachings. Helping others is the goal. That's why those physiognomists who don't understand this grace can't really practice the best physiognomy as a way to benefit others. Also, such physiognomists don't understand that heaven's order is changing day to day, and they will spoil people with their diagnosis. This is fair to say. We have to be really careful.

#3. Japan, China, India — All Are God's Country

Q. Shinto is big, but narrow. We don't talk about it so much. But Taoism, Confucianism, and Buddhism are wide and deep and are talked about by people. What is your opinion?

A. That is a great misunderstanding. Shinto is everywhere, in China, Japan, and India. I can say the mind or heart is God. Bright and clear mind — that we call God. Therefore, Shinto's nature is good, clear, radiant. It is the tao of the great shining God. That grace shines everywhere, all over the universe. This we humans call nature. If we see that clarity in humans, we say it is human nature. That radiance we call Amaterasu Omikami — He Who Shines over the Whole World.[3] He is perfect like a crystal bowl, flawless, completely round. That perfection fills the whole universe. That's why we call him God. God is everywhere, so why am I not divine also?

A man who understands divinity also understand the tao of the world and practices tao well. That's why we say mind is equal to Amaterasu Omikami. He governs all over. That's why the three countries are God's country, where the mind equals God. Not only Japan, but all three countries are God's country. When heaven shines, the tao is to understand God. All three countries are God's countries.

Because Japan is courteous and polite, our starting point is to decide the correct positions. Therefore, even if Japan becomes chaotic and the Emperor's child or grandchild is bad or foolish, still he is respected and the empire continues. China's manner is not so good, but they emphasize wisdom and respect for the tao. If the Emperor's child is foolish in China, he is not allowed to succeed to rule, and a man of lower class who is very smart and follows a clear tao is able to become emperor. Existence of such a genius proves there is divinity. If the tao is shining and clear, that is God's radiance and beauty. Knowing God is the tao for all three countries. Each country has a different name because each one is different, but their origin is the same. God's clear, shining brightness is their origin.

#4 Role of the Three Teachings — Shintoism, Confucianism, Buddhism

Q. If Shinto were perfect, we wouldn't need Confucianism or Buddhism from other countries. But it's because Shinto is not enough, that naturally we are using these other teachings. Don't you think so?

A. We talk about Confucianism and Buddhism, because they are reflections of the same order. The same with Shinto. That's why this country is using all these religions. Since ancient times, these ways of life have always existed in these three countries. Even in Buddhist lands, the countries cannot be managed by only Buddhism's basic philosophy of benevolence or mercy. In Confucian regions, *rei* — order, courtesy, politeness, decourum — alone cannot govern the country.[4] Therefore, in these three countries, it is best to govern with all three teachings. Our country has three major shrines — the Ise-Jingu for Shintoism, the Hachiman-Gu for Buddhism, and the Kasuga-Taisha in Kyoto to worship Confucius.[5] In Japan, Amaterasu-Omikami is the chief deity. Hachiman-Gu is the Buddhist deity. In their ceremony, releasing animals is important. We call that Hachiman Dai Bosatsu. He is a reflection of heaven's order in nature and also loves people to manage the country. Also at the Kasuga Shrine, the Confucianists have a special ceremony for catching birds which ruin farmlands. They sacrifice birds and animals as though they catch demons in order to restore harmony to the country. The Emperor governs on the basis of the law with the aid of the *shin* of the Right and Left.[6] They govern the nation by giving mercy to the people and by catching criminals to restore balance to society. To really make order, all three countries need the three teachings. That is the real origin of Shintoism, Confucianism, and Buddhism.

Amaterasu-Omikami is the God of the Sun. His origin is modesty. That's why if you are modest, you can manage yourself. Kasuga Shrine has small yang *ki* to grow and helps you to climb up and succeed in society. That's why a special ceremony to catch birds is held at the Kasuga Shrine after the winter solstice. Meanwhile, Hachiman-Gu correlates to the end of the *Mats-Yo* yang and helps life to be reborn. Autumn has *ki* that makes everything die out and return to the soil. To compensate for this sorrow, they have a ceremony of Hojyokai in August. This is symbolized by this deity who doesn't want to see all dying. That's why if you keep humble and modest, you will be able to become noble and keep a long life. That is the protective teaching of the Hachiman Shrine.

That's why God is to be found all over. God is living in people's hearts, and in God there is no distinction or rank. Therefore God lives in everyone. That's why traditionally it is said that all deities are the same. They say God comes to a person who is very humble and honest.

Q. In our country, it is said that Amaterasu comes down from heaven above. In India, it is said the gods are standing on the earthly paradise. Why this difference?

A. All gods are born in paradise. They are putting heaven underfoot. Japan is located in the East. It's energy is like morning, when yang starts to rise. India is located in the West. It's energy is more like afternoon, when yang starts to end. That's why Japan's teachings are more yang and India's teachings are more yin. China is between them. Its position is in the center or middle of the flower. If people understand beginning and end, then the teachings of Shinto, Confucianism, and Buddhism are all very clear. That's why if at the beginning and end of life, you become modest and discipline yourself, you are almost one with the tao. Even if your physiognomy is very poor, you will become rich and prosperous. But if your physiognomy is very good and you study such a tao, but yourself are not moderate at the beginning and end and do not discipline yourself, you will use up your wealth and fortune and become poor. That's why if you don't know the order of beginning and end, before and after, later you cannot follow the tao and practice physiognomy. You will not understand good and bad, fortune and misfortune. Such a person we call foolish. They may look like a physiognomist but they are not really. Such persons are just misguiding people and making them wonder. They are like foxes and skunks.

#5 Li Po Was Not Only a Big Drinker

Big Drinkers Don't Become Wise

Q. You have said that if one eats and drinks in a disorderly way, he can't progress. But in the T'ang Dynasty the poet Li Po became very famous for drinking but was renowned as a wise person.[7] I am thinking great people don't need to be modest in eating and drinking. What do you think?

A. If one drinks a lot, his mind automatically becomes chaotic. But in Li Po's case, his mind didn't wobble even after drinking. That is why he became famous. If a small person drinks a lot, his mind automatically becomes disorderly, and he can't do anything. How can he become famous? Li Po could drink more than others, but his mind did not move and he was extraordinary. If Li Po really had drunk too much and became unconscious, nobody would have known his name. Also in our country, Goto Mata-Uemon, a famous samurai, drank more sake than other people with his mind not affected, and that is why he is well known for generations. People think Li Po drank a lot and ate a lot, but actually he may have been humble and modest and in control of himself. Another poet said of Li Po, "100 cups, 100 poems." That means for each cup he drank, he made one poem. I wonder whether he was really a wise man. Rather he simply was gifted in what he liked. It cannot be justified to call him a wise man if he is good at only what he likes. A wise man is the one who influences the world with the tao that he has mastered.

#6 Relief of Terminal Sicknesses with Soft Rice

Because Food and Drink Are Not Orderly, Illness Arises

Q. A sick person asks a question. "Recently, my *hara* has been in pain, day and night. I am experiencing great suffering. I'm still eating as usual, three or four times a day. But I can't do my job. I have searched for and tried many kinds of medicine and prayed to God and Buddha. But there is no cure."

A. You have become sick because of overeating. I can say generally if one's food and drink is not orderly, even with no physiognomic signs of ill health, he is sure to create big sickness. All the illnesses of someone like this are self-created. He is responsible for his own sickness and suffering. Recovery is very slow. Because of not being humble or modest, his sickness cannot be cured, even if he prays to God or Buddha. From now on, if you would like to pray, you firstly should worship God or Buddha by offering them your own food which you have cut down. You can eat three meals a day of soft rice. Such a person can have two bowls at each meal and pray one hundred days. Then you will be able to recover completely. I have tested this in some people with success. Their way of eating and drinking was disorderly, and their sickness arose from stagnated food. That's why I can say for any type of difficult illness, you should be very modest and take only two bowls of soft rice at each meal and practice this for one hundred days to heal. If you have been suffering for several years, you can recover in one year. If you are really modest and orderly about food and drink, you will never become sick. From time to time, as a result of changing seasons of hot or cold weather, you might have to stay in bed, but not for more than three days.

#7 Curing Someone Who Has Lost Their Taste by Eating Less Food

Stagnated Food and Sickness

Q. I have a tendency to have many illnesses. As a result, my food has no taste. How can I restore its taste?

A. Lack of taste does not arise from many sicknesses. It comes from nothing but stagnated food. Firstly, if you don't have an appetite, eat two bowls a day instead of three. If you usually take two bowls, cut back to only one. Anyway, if your stomach is hungry, why cannot you eat and taste? This way, if you eat food moderately, automatically your taste will come back, and stagnated food will not stay in your stomach. If a person doesn't have stagnated food, sickness won't arise. Many sicknesses arise in this way, but there is nothing to say about them because they come from the same origin. Every disease comes from overeating and stagnated, undigested food. Be careful and be modest.

#8 One Who Doesn't Pursue His Ambition Gives No Value to Society

A Person Who Doesn't Pursue Can't Attain

Q. I have changed my job several times but have never been successful. I have several talents in art. Please tell me which is best to follow.

A. In any field you wish to develop or any job you want to follow, you would not find it easy in the beginning because you are impatient. You have to concentrate and put your whole spirit into your work for a couple of years. Then after that, if you become an expert in whatever you are doing, you will understand your work well and be successful. Until now, you couldn't succeed because you have never put your heart and energy into your work. A person like you who changes his mind often is just like a toad in a bamboo basket. In the basket, there appear many exits. The toad decides it is going to go out one exit, and then it suddenly turns around and goes another way without success. It is not really putting its whole effort into getting out from one exit. Its mind is irritated and turns to the right and left. Still, it can't get out, and in the end its energy and spirit are worn out and it dies. You are just like this. You will constantly change your job and suffer and in the end will die unhappily. If someone is very good at controlling his mind, and has steady, even energy, he is like a toad in a box with a tiny hole. The toad finds just one small hole when it looks around to escape. The toad puts its whole effort and energy to reaching that one place and can escape. Even insects and animals have this capacity.

That's why, if as a human being, he puts his mind, heart, and energy together, he can even pass through a big mountain. And if he really concentrates on one thing, we can't say he won't succeed. Because he doesn't try, he can achieve nothing. If he cannot do it, the reason is because he enjoys too much animal food and drinking and has time to fool around. But he can't really put his mind, spirit, and energy into anything. That's why he constantly postpones everything. That's why he is never able to be successful in his job. Then he changes work again and again. His whole life will end in misery.

People who are not moving ahead to accomplish a single thing are valueless for society. Such persons will die unnoticed by people except by friends and neighbors. We call such a death a dog's death. You are just like this. If you don't disagree, take up one job with the spirit of being willing to die for it. Then you certainly will progress. For example, if an enemy is surrounding someone from ten directions and he tries to fight in all ten directions, then he will immediately be defeated and killed. But even if a few million men or houses surround him, if he really concentrates, not minding to die and fighting in only one direction, he is able to pass through and escape. It's the same strategy in any field. That's why you must go in one direction and put your whole life's effort into it. Otherwise you can't understand the tao.

#9 The Three Teachings of Shintoism, Confucianism, and Buddhism Have No Borderlines Between Them

Q. When you are alive, you have physiognomic signs. After death, they don't exist. I think physiognomy therefore is based on Shintoism. But, Sensei, you are always worshipping Buddha. I think this is a mistake.

A. I don't know how Shinto, Confucianism, and Buddhism differ. They are very clear and return to the one. That's why I just worship heaven and earth and respect everything. In Shinto, it's said that everything is *Konton* or chaos and confusion.[8] In Confucianism, they talk about *Mei Toku* or clear virtue.[9] In Buddhism, they call it *Mida* Buddha.[10] *Mida* comes from *Konton. Konton* comes from *Mei Toku. Mei Toku* comes from *Mida.* All are one, and there is no difference.

Also, if someone can really see from their heart the whole order of creation — the grace of millions and trillions of things — they are not just Buddhists. In each different Buddhist sect, they worship Amida. In Sanskrit, "A" stands for the ten different directions. The sound of "A" and the character of "A" belong to heaven. "Mi" belongs to the human world and means helping everything. "Da" belongs to earth. The character of "mi" stands for eight thousand things. That's why we can say heaven, man, and earth. Everything is in Amida. That's why the character of "Ah" shines in the ten directions. The character of "mi" serves everyone. "Da" represents the eight hundred thousand things on earth which are helped. Also all society and hundreds of thousands of things start from "A." Then from "da" they start to grow. Then through "mi," they intermix and help each other. "Mi" means every phenomena. Everything arises like this. Also every person and everything grows in the soil — in earth. In Buddhism, we call the structure of this earth *Jodo* or paradise. Everything lives on this wonderful earth. That's why we can say humans and all things are *mida.* Buddha itself, *konton* and *mei toku* have the same origin. That's why if you are not humble, spoil your body, and waste many things it is just like destroying *mida.*

On the other hand, if you honor the myriads of beings, don't spoil or waste things, and take care of everything very well, naturally the body of such persons will become like the Nyorai Buddha.[11] Our body is the individual Buddha. Also fortune and misfortune follow whatever you wish to do. Your mind creates the appearance and disappearance of phenomena. That's why we say spiritual paradise follows the mind. For the tao of someone like this is to see Buddha — without thinking or meditating. At the end, he discovers *mida* for himself. Then truly from his heart, he understands countless phenomena and the value of all things. That's why they are never extravagant. He always wears modest clothing, takes humble meals, and day to day accumulates grace. His grace grows and permeates society. Even if such a person lives on a mountain or in a cave, everyone will be aware of his grace and honor him. This call comes about as a result of what he's done, from his moderation. Because of this, he becomes *mida*. Then his light brightens and extends in all directions.

Meanwhile, if you don't understand heaven and earth's grace and are always extravagant, disorderly, and wasting things, it as if you are destroying that Buddha you have inside yourself. Such persons decorate themselves gorgeously on the outside, but nobody would employ these people. They spoil their own virtues and suffer a lot because they don't understand heaven and earth's order.

But the other way, of course, our human knowledge and emotions change together along with with millions of phenomena. One can purify this changing intellect or emotion. Then if he understands the law of order, he can discover Buddha or real wisdom. He can discover Buddha within himself — attain enlightenment or become Buddha. For my teaching of physiognomy, the origin or center is the personal Buddha. This is the beginning. Once you understand this tao, you can explain this way to help society. That is the target.

B. Animal Food Disturbs the Mind

Q. People who love and eat a lot of animal food have unclear minds. I'm always eating animal food, but my mind is not cloudy. Does eating animal food always make anyone's mind — including upper and lower class persons — cloudy?

A. It's really true that animal food makes the mind cloudy.

That's why after eating, the mind is not really clear and clean. After eating vegetables, the mind automatically becomes clear. That's why someone who doesn't eat animal food we call *Sei Shi*.[12] Also *Sei shin* means clear mind.

Anyone noble or low class, if his mind is cloudy, finds it difficult to understand tao. With unclear mind, he can't manage himself. That's why Buddhist monks ask people not to eat animal food on certain days so that people can understand the tao of Buddhism. If the mind is clear and clean, it can't engage in bad conduct and people can control themselves more. Even when one has to eat meat, if he is very modest and eats a very small amount of animal food, his mind stays clear. But food and drink for ordinary people are usually very difficult to control. Unless he determines to be almost a monk, it is very difficult to be modest. If someone really wants to become moderate, that means his mind *ki* is clear and clean. This is the essence of managing yourself. That's why someone who leaves his ego to discipline himself is a true Buddhist. True Buddhists don't engage in bad conduct and are always modest in their food.

On the other hand, if one understands his limitations, and eats a small amount of animal food accordingly, his mind is clear. Therefore, naturally he would not eat much. But if he doesn't know his limitations, he eats too much and his mind will become cloudy. In general, ordinary people limit their food, but if they see animal food, their appetite increases and without knowing it they eat a lot. Meat eating really makes their mind cloudy. If a person has a really clear mind, he is very careful and orderly when they cook, but someone with a cloudy mind will cut vegetables and cook in a very disorderly way. They say: "Somone who has mastered himself doesn't eat unclean food. And if the way of cooking is not clear and clean, they will not eat what is prepared for them." That shows that ancient people also talked about the order of food and drink. Really I can say food could make the mind cloudy.

C. What Is True Inheritance?

Q. I would like to leave my children and grandchildren prosperous and bequeath to them my house and wealth. Am I am capable of doing so in my life?

A. What you want to do is very bad and is not a parent's benevolence. For children, inheritance is very, very bad, like an enemy. If parents intend to leave a child wealth, he will always be thinking of that. He spends his time idly month by month, day by day and does not put his effort into his work. He will end up losing the house and family line. If parents really wish their offspring to become wealthy and continue endlessly, they must first be honest all the time and show that to their children. And for children and offspring, they must not waste even a small item. Practicing these virtues is the thing parents must leave for their progeny and for their house. Then for thousands of generations, their house's fortune will not change and their name will never end. If parents are keeping modesty as their family custom and giving it to their descendents to keep the family, they will be worthy of their ancestors' great efforts and bequeath their great love.

#10 Anyone Who Has More Than One Year of Life Left Can Extend His Longevity

Food Is the Origin of Wealth, Happiness, and Longevity

Q. I am in early old age now, but have not been able to manage my life well. From now on, I'd like to control myself and realize *fukurokuju* or wealth, happiness, and longevity.[13] Do you think I will be able to manage by being humble and modest?

A. If one has less than one year of life left, it's very difficult to extend his life. If he has only one year left, he will be able to extend his life another year by being very modest for a year. If he has been modest for ten years, he can extend his life another ten years. Happiness and wealth automatically follow. I can say that our life exists in heaven. Our food and wealth exist on earth. We only receive these *fukorokuju* — wealth, happiness, and longevity. Whether they are noble or poor, everybody has wealth, happiness, and longevity. There is no one who doesn't have these at birth. Life is eternal and cannot be measured. But wealth and food have limits. That's why everyone from the Emperor to ordinary people must observe their limitations of food. Generally, we say the standard quantity is three to five *go* of food per day. People who eat more than this or who waste food are definitely destroying their wealth, happiness, and longevity. That's why someone who is a big eater is never able to progress in society and become famous, and their life is short.

On the other hand, if somone is modest in food, he will become wealthy, happy, and enjoy a long life. He is able to keep *fukorokuju*. That's why someone who eats a small amount stays healthy and enjoys a certain amount of happiness with only few sicknesses. Happiness and wealth belong to and are fulfilled in society and the world. If they stop at you, you are happy and wealthy. But you cultivate and nourish longevity. The way you nourish longevity determines whether your life is long or short. Life itself is neither long nor short. *Fukurokuju* depends on modesty of food and drink. We talk about life, but life doesn't exist without eating. That's why if one doesn't waste his food, he is able to keep longevity, happiness, and wealth.

That's why we can say food is the origin of human beings. Eating is the beginning. If the origin is chaotic, nothing can be controlled. That's why if someone eats disorderly, his mind becomes chaotic and he can't control his body. Also if one cannot nourish himself properly, he will not be able to manage his home or relate to his wife and children. They too will become disorderly, and his family will end up very dark and unhappy. That's why if you really want to keep wealth, happiness, and longevity, foremost you have to be strict concerning food by cutting down the amount you eat yourself, offering it to heaven, and praying for wealth, happiness, and longevity. I can really say that food is the essence of wealth, happiness, and longevity. That's why if someone is disorderly, extravagant, and foolish in his way of eating, he has lost the essence of life and can't keep wealth, happiness, and longevity.

Q. If what you are saying is true, is gold and silver and those precious treasures not more valuable than food?

A. Because we eat, we can keep our life. Without life, how can we honor our parents? That's why in the whole world, the most important thing is food. After being given life, what he receives is food. That's why a fetus in the mother's womb eats food from the mother who then had morning sickness. We say that the mother is craving what the baby is craving. After birth until the end of life, people eat. When his food ends, life ends, and he dies. That's why even sick people approaching death still like to eat. People bring them food, they eat it up, and then return to their origin. Therefore, if one eats too much, even one mouthful too much, he will spoil his wealth, happiness, and longevity. That's why I conclude that the essence of physiognomy has nothing to do with fortune or misfortune. Destiny is decided entirely by food. Sometimes, signs of current fortune or misfortune, or such minor things, appear in the facial color. But for the direction of our whole life, that is governed by food and drink, whether he eats a big or small amount and is modest and humble. That's why please keep food and drink humble. That is the essence to keep wealth, happiness, and longevity. Really without this, no fortune or misfortune exists.

#11 Physiognomists Who Don't Understand the Origin of Fortune and Misfortune Are Thieves

A. The Essence of Seeing Structure in Physiognomy

Q. One of the disciples came to question and asked what the most important quality was to master physiognomy.

A. Nothing but food and drink. Do not strain your eyes reading texts and books. If you would like to be able to tell fortune and misfortune in physiognomy clearly, I always keep saying do not waste food and drink. Strictly control yourself and understand that you are destroying heaven's life by wasting things. Think that way and decide for yourself that even the smallest amount you will not waste. If one acts like this for three years, then he can clearly discover heaven's order. I'm always practicing like this. I perceive the signs of fortune and misfortune from nature in the person and taste these for myself. Then I advise people. That is really the physiognomist's way of life. If some physiognomist does not do this, he doesn't see people clearly and doesn't understand the origin of fortune and misfortune. He is a a thief of physiognomy. That's why when diagnosing other people, just be modest and humble.

B. The Reason Why Some Stingy People Become Rich

Q. Many times someone who is not modest and humble, but stingy, becomes rich. Does that mean modesty and humility are not necessary?

A. There are some people without modesty and humbleness in their life who create wealth and happiness. Those persons all are stingy. They not only cut down their quantity of food, giving up what they want to eat, but also they give little food for their family. But still someone like this doesn't eat very much himself as a result of his stinginess. He extends that saved food to heaven and earth. Without knowing, he is accumulating heaven's grace and extending his life. For each grain saved, thousands of grains again come back into his life. That's why he is able to get rich. On account of his stinginess, cutting back his family's food seems bad in itself, but wealth is extended to heaven, and eventually the other family members will become more prosperous. People complain about stinginess, but because it is virtuous to heaven and earth, the stingy can progress.

These people tend to be somewhat empty in their physiognomy, and even with hard work it is harder to accumulate wealth and fortune compared with attaining it by being modest and humble.

Heaven and earth originated from nothingness. Yin and yang came into existence, and through that *ki* energy of yin and yang human beings were created. *Ki* energy is primary. Our body is secondary. That's why when you talk about physiognomy, first talk about *ki* energy. Wealth, poverty, happiness, sadness, long life, short life, suffering, and joy are created by our own *ki* energy. The origin of all phenomena is energy. That's why yin and yang — those two energies — are *mei-toku*, bright shining grace, to my way of physiognomy.[14] I don't know the definition of *mei-toku* in Confucian thought.

In heaven and earth, *ki* energy is found everywhere. Therefore, there is nowhere *mei-toku* is not filled. *Mei-toku* never goes away from anyone even for a split second. It it so great that we can't see it with the physical eye. The study of physiognomy starts with *mei-toku* followed by managing oneself.

There is no phenomena which doesn't show physiognomy.[15]

That's why physiognomists should understand the order of all phenomena — heaven and earth. To study and master that is the starting point. Then the goal is to spread the teaching to people and put your effort into accumulating grace for society.

I can say heaven and earth's grace govern every phenomenon's balance of yin and yang. In the beginning, you need to study and understand this. This is a wonderful, great, endless adventure. Also, don't count your profit or reward but accumulate virtue to heaven and earth. A physiognomist who clearly understands grace will become a superior physiognomist and become great and famous. Virtue, *toku*, is also reward (*toku*).[16]

Your virtue becomes heaven and earth's grace, and it will produce gain. Unless you accumulate your virtue, where can you get any gain from? Forgetting about any gain to yourself, you gain if you receive heaven and earth's grace. If you forget heaven and earth's grace and try to get gain for yourself, you can gain nothing. Such persons are all enemies of heaven and earth.

That's why a physiognomist of virtue will never be poor. The only origin of human beings is *mei-toku*. I can say *mei*, sun and moon, belongs to our father and mother. We are born from our parents' grace. All of our body and mind is therefore *mei-toku*. If we don't destroy our body, then it is clear that the source of everything is this radiant energy. All phenomena are born from the grace of the sun and moon. That's why the source of everything is *mei-toku*. All human beings are receiving this energy which nourishes our body and spirit. Beyond the grace of sun and moon, there is nothing more precious. To understand this clearly is all in your hands.

Also, *mei* — yin and yang — is just like king and subject. As yin follows yang, subject follows king. That is the origin. If one doesn't follow this order, his light will not shine clearly. Wife is yin. That's why she follows her husband. If yin and yang match and balance harmoniously, that is the *mei-toku* of heaven and earth. And also human beings are the masters of all phenomena, and from beginning to end should make this order clear. If you understand and observe this, then you will understand *mei-toku* clearly.

This is clearly the tao for the world. Day by day, it's really true. I can say the world's tao is low in the southeast and high in the northwest. Water runs from high to low. This is the *mei-toku* of heaven and earth. Also mountains are high and hundreds of trees are growing on them. The ocean is low and receiving drops of water from the grace of the mountains. That means their *ki* is flowing through. All these accord with the *mei-toku* of heaven and earth. This is the tao of physiognomy. Nothing odd varies from this path. Anything odd is not tao. Everything is clear. That is the tao of physiognomy.

Also my way of physiognomy deals with all phenomena. From beginning to end, I take into account the renewal of all things. The new is the beginning. Things have a beginning, then they have an end. Day by day, they are renewed. That's why day by day we perceive fortune and misfortune and discover one's life's good and bad sides. By observing phenomena, we can know *mu*, nothingness.[17] With a knowledge of *mu*, we can understand all phenomena. From *mu*, all phenomena are created. This process continues day to day, not stopping for even a second. Also the circulating of blood and energy in the body flows just like this. The facial color also follows this course. Further, the meaning of renewal is like cutting down a tree with an axe. Because the tree was growing in the beginning, in the end it will be cut down. If something is born to be useful in the beginning, it will be returned to the soil in the end. Then it will be reborn, just like food cycling and recycling. All phenomena are reborn in this way. If you don't perceive this, you can't diagnose people. If you understand that all phenomena are always changing and newly born, then you understand that all people are always new too.

Everyone has different limits. Some people are worth a thousand *koku* of rice, others ten thousand. Each person has a different limit. Everyone is helping others. If he has no subjects, how can one call a lord a lord? Nobody would honor him. That's why the lord's grace all can be judged by his subjects. That's why a lord caring for people is just like parents taking care of their children. We say that you make each subject reborn day by day. That you should do daily. The Emperor has four different kinds of people, and each of these people has his own subjects, who perhaps are his wife and children. If you are a widow, then all people are your people. From the Emperor down to ordinary people, all phenomena serve human beings. That's why we say people are master of all things. Even the widow treats all phenomena just like servants to conduct daily life. Even for the lowest grade people, everything used — for example, a bowl or a torn cloth — is their subject. All people are nourished by many things and conduct various things. What nourishes and helps me are these subjects and thousands of materials. Take care of all materials just as your lord and parent. If you take care of them really well, you are refreshing your people. If you treat them as new day by day, we say that you are recreating *mei-toku*, the clear, shining beginning of the universe.

If a physiognomist doesn't understand this order, he can't understand heaven's clear shining order in phenomenal reality. If he is not clear and doesn't understand where he is standing, he can't diagnose others. If you would like to practice physiognomy of the world, you must understand *mei-toku*, the universal virtue and compassion of physiognomy. Then you will find out the tao of society. If you would like to diagnose everything under heaven, you should clearly understand *mei-toku*. One who knows the tao of society knows his limitations and can stand within them. A person who fails to understand this order is disorderly, foolish, and becomes arrogant. People like this who diagnose others can't influence society. If you clearly observe order in your own life and help other people understand the tao in their life, that is the best virtue of all. If your life is not resting on this foundation, you can't guide people for the better. Also you are blind and can't give light to others. Rather you spoil them. Abiding within your limits is virtue, and you will be able to manage everything well. But if a person doesn't respect his limits, badness will develop and he will never be bright but dark. That's why for understanding human destiny, if you are orderly, then the whole of life, including fortune and misfortune, will become very clear to you. Some elders said, "People should be content to be steady within the limits, and not look around. One who doesn't stay within is not right. He will miss the return of heaven's fortune." You can catch fortune from heaven if you stay in one place when it comes to you, so that you can make things right.

In the end, when the cycle is complete, heaven's yang departs, but if one waits, it will come back again. Then he can start to make things right again. That's why in any tao, one who stops within and stays eventually masters the tao, and he can manage the house easily. Unless a physiognomist stays within this great virtue, he can't understand nature's order. One who doesn't understand nature's order is of no use for society. He is more foolish than bamboo or wood.

The essence of my teaching can't be written in a book. Number one, be humble and modest. Then learn to observe the invisible world, *mu*. You can end your training by finding the order of the universal creation.

I have many students, but few truly can follow this way. Many times, students start the training but don't respect their limitations and give up. That's why I started, set up a curriculum, and charged tuition to teach. But people are disrespecting order and even soiling my reputation. From now on, I don't want to teach my way of diagnosis any more. If there is someone who would really like to train himself, he should find the limit of his stomach and realize that all phenomena are serving him. Then he will be able to master my way of diagnosis. I have been practicing this tao for many years. I have nothing else to teach.

Notes

Introduction

1. Mochi is pounded sweet rice that was traditionally eaten in Japan on New Year's, holidays, and other special occasions.
2. The Tao is the way of heaven and earth, the order of the universe, yin and yang, or what Mizuno calls the "Good Way of Humanity."

Book I

1. Contemporary reports of longevity often stress the person's modest way of eating. According to a recent news item, Mr. Chokichi Hirukawa in Ota City in northern Japan, at age 97, manages to look after his rice paddy and thirty-five mulberry trees without any machines. The farmer eats brown rice or udon noodles, with a little pickles, miso soup, kombu, and beans. He chews very well and stops eating when his stomach is 80 percent full. He enjoys a cup of sake every evening.
2. In traditional Far Eastern medicine, signs of approaching death included: lack of power and light in the eyes, a pale color, crying over sadness and difficulties, a contracted tongue, a mouth shut tight and lack of talking, a black color or vibration on the outside of the ear, short temper, inability to complete sentences while talking, a blue/green line on the nose, and a black line from the back of the neck to the ear.
4. The study of these influences was traditionally known as Nine Star Ki in the Far East. Because of changing atmospheric and climactic conditions, it was believed that traveling in certain directions at different times could have a beneficial or harmful effect.
5. The hara [腹] is the center of the intestinal area below the navel and governs digestion, decompositon, and absorption of food, water, and energy as well as body equilibrium and overall vitality.
6. In those days, family was very important. The family house, business, wealth, etc. were inherited by the eldest son. No son meant the end of the family name. The family would then either find a husband for the daughter or adopt a man who could keep the family name going.

7. In Shinto and Buddhism, it is customary to offer some food in front of the family altar for the spirits of those who have died.

8. [福] (riches, wealth, *fuku*) is pronounced the same as [覆] (decline, *fuku*).

9. The opening line of the *Heike Monogatari* (Tale of the Heike), a famous anthology of medieval Japanese poetry.

10. The five grains were rice, buckwheat, millet, barley, and aduki bean (though not a grain classified as such).

11. Rice was measured in [石], *koku*, and *koku* was the usual term for wealth.

12. Samurai customarily ate twice a day, but when fighting five times.

13. Such a samurai is expected to inherit his father's position.

14. The salary was measured and given in rice.

15. In Buddhism, a Bodhisattva is someone who postpones his or her own happiness to serve others.

16. These refer to old coins. One sen [銭], the smallest, was made of copper.

17. In Japan, someone with mental illness was said to be possessed by the spirit of a fox or a badger. In modern society, this condition is known as schizophrenia.

18. In Oriental medicine, excess and deficiency are known as *jitsu* [実] and *kyo* [虚], and sickness can be traced to excess or deficiency of *ki* in one or more organs and systems.

19. There are certain traditional ages when one is said to encounter difficulties, including from 0 to 3 and from 41 to 43.

20. Respecting parents and elders was one of the Confucian virtues.

21. [殺生戒], *sessnokai*, or the observance of non-killing, is the rule, and monks are not allowed to take any life.

22. Karma is the law of cause and effect or natural order.

23. Described at length later in this Book and in Book 2.

24. In traditional Chinese physiognomy, signs of a violent, excessively yang nature, included: very flat forehead and back, short and widespread cheeks, big and bulging eyes or big and sunken eyes, intense, strong eyes, big, wide nose, big, crooked mouth, very big and strong chin, and high cheeks. Such people have a tendency to kill, commit arson, rape, commit bad behavior, rob and assault others, attack with a knife, and steal. Signs of a disorderly, yin structure are: long and dark face, small and flat forehead, eyes half open or piercing, nostrils uneven, and often flat, crooked mouth, uneven teeth, and square chin. Such people have a tendency to rob, steal, lie, deceive, make false contracts, and take other people's property and land.

25. Children are expected to pray for their parents' spirits and tend their altars. Dying before one's parents violates natural law.

26. "House" could be replaced with "family." But in the Orient, the word *house* is used in these cases, i.e., the house's reputation over some generations is more important than that of the families that constitute it.

27. A *to* [斗] equals 18.05 liters or 19.04 quarts.

28. This is a play on paper [紙], pronounced *kami*, and deity [神], also pronounced *kami* and meaning righteous and clear.

29. In the Far East, contracts do not carry signatures but the seal or stamp of

each party.

30. *Go* [碁] is the ancient game of strategy played with 361 white and black stones. *Shogi* [将棋] is Japanese-style chess.

31. Geomancy was the traditional art of understanding household arrangement, environmental influences, and personal or social destiny.

32. Fire [火], *hi*, is pronounced the same as day [日] *hi*.

Book II

1. In Buddhism there are five kinds of bad wives: those who are proud of their beauty and style, those proud of their (maiden) family's wealth, those who boast how hard they do housework, those who boast how hard they take care of the children, and those who improperly use psychic power and energy.

2. *Mandokoro* [政所] = governor.

3. In ancient Chinese fortune-telling, the directions and their attributes are: 1) North, wife, make solid, foundation; 2) South, husband, becoming loose, lazy, power; 3) East, child, progress, activity; 4) West, old man, shrink, preparation; 5) Northeast, husband's lover, immature wife; 6) Southeast, young man, between child and husband; 7) Southwest, yin man, between old man and husband; and 8) Northwest, Geisha, old woman.

4. *Kitanokata* = [北の方], a person in the North.

5. *Midaidokoro* = [御台所] Respectful Base Place; this word is now used fo the kitchen.

6. *Okugate* = [奥方], a person at the (deep) back.

7. A traditional Buddhist sutra, *Hanya-Shin-Gyo*.

8. A traditional saying of Confucius.

9. Taoism is also called [道教], "Five *To* Rice Tao," because anyone can go and learn by giving five *to* of rice. Taoism includes teaching special medicine for longevity, dietetics, and self-massage.

10. Traditional Chinese medicine recommended wheat be eaten in spring, rice in summer, buckwheat in autumn, mochi in winter, and millet between seasons.

11. *Ho-Jo* = [放生].

12. *Dhyani* comes from *dhyana*, Sanskrit, for "meditation," which in Japanese is pronounced as *Zen*.

13. The then capital of Japan.

14. *Go* = [合], old Japanese measurement = 0.180 liter or 0.32 pint.

15. *Gaki* = [餓鬼], demons or inhabitans of the inferno of hunger, classed beneath human beings in Buddhism.

16. At that time wheat was regarded as the grain of poor peasants.

17. *Okara* is the soy pulp left over from making tofu. It is edible and used in macrobiotic cooking.

18. Refined rice, polished about 50 percent, started to prevail among rich city people from the mid-Edo period.

19. A rook is a large bird.

20. According to legend, a phoenix lives on cold water.

21. In those days, Buddhism as a national religion was very powerful and re-

ceived lots of donations and sometimes sold and lent money.

22. The Honganji sect is a major branch of Jodo Shin Shu Buddhism.

23. The founder of the Jodo Shin sect of Pure Land Buddhism Shinran (1173-1263), went to a temple at age nine, became a student of Honen at 29, traveled around Japan from age 39, and preached until his death.

24. In feudal Japan, employees customarily lived in the household.

25. The Angry Buddha.

26. The original measure was one *go*, about a cup. See Book 2, Note 16.

27. Traditional Confucian teachings stress cultivating the five virtues (*Go-Jo*) [仁義礼智信] of the mind. They are 1) Kindness (*Jin*); 2) Truth (*Gi*); 3) Righteousness (*Rei*); 4) Respect for Parents and Children (*Chi*); and 5) Wisdom (*Shin*).

28. *Jyo butsu* [成仏] = to die, return to, to become Buddha. There is an old Buddhist belief that anyone except a serious criminal becomes a Buddha after death.

29. The name of a Buddhist sutra.

20. The tiger's face and the bull's horns make a demon. The monkey's face and sheep's horns also make a demon.

31. *Hokke-kyo* is the Japanese name for the *Lotus Sutra*, one of the chief texts of Mahayana Buddhism.

Book III

1. In Hamamatsu, Oritaro Shimizu, the silk-weaving manufacturer who borrowed money after World War II from poor rice farmers to pay for Aveline's ticket to the United States, was a disciple of Amaterasu, the Sun Goddess. On a recent visit to Japan, we visited him, and at age 95, he taught us a special chant to Amaterasu that can lead to long life: "The heavenly shining sun is our ancestral life and my life. You are my father and mother."

2. *O sei seki zur* is a medicinal remedy made from the lily and other wild flowers, grasses, and roots. It is cooked like mochi. Eating one small ball every day will change white hair to black.

3. The Japanese words [仙人] *sennin* or [神仙] *shinsen*, comes from the Chinese *xianren* or *hsien-jen*, an immortal. We have translated it as a free man (or woman). A free man traditionally lived in the mountains and through a period of self-education attained health, happiness, and peace. The *sennin* mastered their desires by studying the Order of the Universe, attained longevity, often one hundred years or more, came down to the fields to help people or taught and practiced healing, and practiced alchemy. In the mountains, where grain did not grow, they customarily lived on pine needles, nuts, bark, roots, mountain vegetables, and mushrooms. Before civilization spread several hundred years ago, they lived in the mountains of Japan, China, India, and other parts of the East.

4. Oshu is located in northern Japan.

5. The Chinese title is *Retsu Sen Den* or "Free Man's Textbook."

6. The Three Lights are stars in the Big Dipper.

7. *So O Zan* [相王山] means Physiognomy King of the Mountain.

8. *Namboku Do* [南北道] means Temple of North and South.

9. *Namboku An* [南北庵] means Priest's Chapel of North and South.

10. *Nanbokuji* [南北寺] means Temple of North and South.

11. *Kagiya Kumataro* [鍵屋の熊太郎] means Keymaker Bear Boy.

12. *Mizuno Syumei* [水野主圭] means Master of the Water Field.

13. *Mizuno Namboku* [水野南北] means Waterfield of the North and South.

14. Karma is the law of cause and effect. In Japanese, karma is known as [因果] *inga*.

15. In old Chinese physiognomy, signs of loneliness included: 1) a square hand, 2) overly thick eyebrows, 3) overly high nose, 4) big and fat ear (for a woman), 5) ends of mouth drooping, 6) short lower lip, 7) round forehead (for a woman), 8) knotty finger joints, 9) skin below the eyes hanging down (in a man), 10) dark skin below or around the eyes (in a woman).

16. *Tenmoku* [天目] = valuable plates or bowls.

17. *Go ki* [御器] = five dishes or bowls.

18. Nanki Moku Jiki Shonin was a famous Buddhist holy priest in Kumano, who ate ate only mountain roots and tree fruits.

19. Jodo Shin Shu Buddhism is based on the teachings of Shinran. See Book 2, Notes 22-23.

20. The sake referred to here is not ordinary sake but sake in which animal food or herbs have been added for strength.

21. According to Mizuno, signs of a good woman include: 1) a round head, flat forehead, 2) thin bones, with soft muscles, 3) dark hair and pink/red mouth, 4) large eyes, good eyebrows, 5) thin fingers, soft hand, 6) small voice, but clear and with a sound fresh like running water, 7) showing no teeth when laughing, 8) when walking, feet and toes facing inside, 9) when sitting, appearing full like a flower, and 10) a clean mind, kind, with a good clean smell of the skin.

22. *Un mei* [運命] = fortune life, or the good fortune of being alive.

23. *Hito* [火止] = fire.

24. *To do maru* [止] = staying inside.

25. *Hi i* [火去] = death.

26. *Un ten* [運転] = turning fortune; *un-sen* [運旋] = expanding fortune; and *un-do* [運動] = returning fortune.

27. *Un sei* [運勢] = moving greatly.

28. *Un ki* [運気] = the power or energy of life. See Note 22 above for *un-mei*.

29. *Go zo* [五臓], the five transformation organs, include the liver and gallbladder, heart and small intestine, spleen-pancreas and stomach, lungs and large intestine, and kidney and bladder.

30. *Un-ki* [運気] means fortune-energy. See Note 28 above.

31. *Go jyo* [五行] = the five transformations or stages of energetic change that all phenomena go through: 1) upward energy, 2) active energy, 3) stabilizing energy, 4) gathering energy, and 5) floating energy. Sometimes they are associated with tree, fire, soil, metal, and water, but it should be understood that these phases or states are dynamic and everchanging, not fixed and immutable.

32. The *ki* of mind or heart in Chinese medicine means activity/power/energy of the heart. Also mental activity of the mind.

33. Leaving animals, see Book 2

34. Cutting is a direct translation. In this text it means cooking properly.

35. The tanden or hara is located below the navel. It is also called the ocean of *ki* energy in acupuncture. In Oriental medicine, it is a good point for treatment of neurosis, hysteria, manic-depression, and schizophrenia.

36. The *san ko* [三甲] is located on the back

37. The *san shin* [三壬] is located on the ankle.

38. [心火] = fire of mind.

39. Ohshu is located in northeast Japan.

Book IV

1. Sorai Ogyu (1666-1728) was a leading Confucian thinker of the Edo period and adviser to two shoguns. Syundai Daza (1680-1747) was a Confucian scholar who excelled in political economy.

2. Kuni-Toko-Tachi-No-Mikoto was a Shinto deity.

3. Amaterasu is the Shinto Sun God or Goddess and mythical ancestor of the imperial family.

4. [礼] or *rei* = order, virtue, reason in Confucian thought.

5. Ise *Jingu* or shrine is one of the most important Shinto shrines. It is located in the city of Ise in Mie Prefecture and enshrines the ancestral gods of the imperial family. The Inner Shrine is dedicated to Amaterasu. Hachiman, originally a Shinto deity who protected warriors, came to be viewed as a protector of Buddhism. The *Gu* or shrine to Hachiman was established in Kyoto in 859 and patronized by the Minamoto family and other warrior clans during the middle ages. Kasuga Shrine, sacred to Shinto, is located in Nara where it was founded in 709 to protect the new capital city. Its unique architecture and deer that roam freely around the temple precincts continue to attract many people today.

6. *Shin* [臣] of the Right and Left were traditional officials of state who advised the ruler.

7. Li Po (701-762), a Chinese poet and wanderer, is one of the most famous poets in Chinese history.

8. *Konton* [混沌] = chaos or confusion.

9. *Mei-toku* [明徳] = clear virtue.

10. Mida or Amida Buddha is the Buddha of Boundless Light (Sanskrit, *Amitabha*). Amida is reversed especially by the Pure Land sect which emphasizes chanting his name as a spiritual practice.

11. Nyorai was the Buddha's appelation for himself. It is the Japanese translation of the Sanskrit *Tathagata*, "thus come," or the one who has come from or gone to truth.

12. *Sei* [精] means rice and green and *Shin* means God. Together *sei shin* [精神] means spiritual. Another meaning is "clear mind."

13. *Fukorokuju* [福禄寿] means wealth, happiness, and longevity.

14. *Mei-toku* [明徳], see Note 9.

15. The word for physiognomy in Japanese is [人相学] formed from the ideographs for eye and tree.

16. Toku [徳] means virtue or reward.

17. Mu [無] = nothingness.

Glossary

Amaterasu Omikami "He or She Who Shines Over the Whole World," a principal divinity in Shinto mythology, commonly known as the Sun Goddess.

Bodhisattva "Enlightenment being," one who has vowed to become a Buddha or realized Buddha nature and returned to the world to help others. A Bodhisattva is a person who guides others with a deep understanding of yin and yang.

Buddha "Awakened one," a person who has attained universal understanding and spirit. Sakyamuni (also known as Siddartha Gautama), the historical Buddha, lived in northern India in the 6th century B.C.

Confucius The Chinese philosopher and sage who lived in the 6th century B.C. and had a deep understanding of yin and yang.

Directionology The theory that the cardinal directions influence human affairs. In the Far East, this is also known as *Nine Star Ki* and derives from the *I Ching* and teachings of the ancient spiritual world.

Edo The old name for Tokyo, which became the capital of Japan during the Meiji Era. Also the period of Japanese history from 1615-1868.

Five transformations The five stages of energy that characterize all pheonomena: *upward, active, downward, condensing,* and *floating* energy. Often these are translated as *tree, fire, soil, metal,* and *water,* but the five stages should be viewed dynamically rather than as fixed states.

Fukurokuju "Wealth, happiness, and longevity," the property of all life.

Geomancy The art of household placement, building siting, and city and country planning according to yin and yang and *Nine Star Ki.*

Hara Energy center located deep in the intestines below the navel, also known as the *tanden.*

Heart Sutra A Buddhist sutra known in Sanskrit as Prajna Paramita Hridaya and in Japanese as Hanya Hamarmita Shingyo, expressing the heart or essence of the teachings of the Buddha on the Order of the Universe.

Hidden virtue In Mizuno's physiognomy, there are two types of virtue or grace. *Yin toku* is good deeds, thoughts, or donation that are done in private without calling attention to oneself. *Yang toku* is right action that is done in public or which is noticed by others.

Ho-Jo "Releasing life," the Buddhist practice of collecting or purchasing live birds, fish, and other animals and setting them free.

Ise Shrine The national shrine in southeast Japan dedicated to Amaterasu and the Goddess of Food and Agriculture.

Ki The natural electromagnetic energy of heaven and earth that carries energy and consciousness to the meridians, chakras, and cells.

Kuni-Toko-Tachi-No-Mikoto In Shinto mythology, the first deity born after the creation of heaven and earth.

Kyoto The capital of Japan during the time which Mizuno lived, a beautiful city of ten thousand Buddhist temples.

Mei toku The grace of sun and moon, the clear shining source of life.

Meiji Era The period of modern Japanese history that began in 1868 and ended in 1912.

Miso Fermented paste with a sweet taste and salty flavor made from soybeans, usually barley or rice, and sea salt. Used in soup and as a seasoning.

Mochi A cake or dumpling made from cooked, pounded sweet rice. In Japan, mochi is traditionally eaten on New Year's and other special occasions.

Mu "Nothingness," the immaculate world out of which the phenomenal world arose and to which it will return.

Myo The invisible spirit or beauty in all phenomena.

Ohsawa, George The founder of modern macrobiotics (1893-1966) was born in Japan and traveled and taught in Europe, Asia, Africa, and North America.

Oriental astrology In the Far East, the signs of the zodiac are: Rat (January), Ox (February), Tiger (March), Rabbit (April), Dragon (May), Serpent

(June), Horse (July), Sheep (August), Monkey (September), Cock (October), Dog (November), Boar (December).

Physiognomy The art of judging character or destiny according to the features of the face or body. Mizuno defines it further as a way of life, leading to endless spiritual realization.

Reincarnation The universal cycle of life, especially the idea of successive rebirths in various bodies from one lifetime to the next.

Sake Wine made from fermented rice.

Samurai Member of the traditional warrior class in Japan.

Seaweed An edible sea vegetable such as *kombu, wakame, hiziki,* and *nori.*

Sennin "Free man [or woman]," a sage who lived in the mountains of Japan and was said to have discovered the secrets of immortality.

Shinto "The Way of the Gods," the traditional way of life of Japan. Amaterasu and Susa-no-wo-no-mikoto are principal divinities.

Shogun The powerful military leader of Japan who ruled, often from behind the scenes, in the name of the Emperor.

Soba Noodles made from buckwheat flour combined with whole wheat.

Tao "The Way" of heaven and earth, the endless cycle of yin and yang. The term also refers to a spiritual practice or art such as the tao of painting, the tao of woodworking, the tao of physiognomy.

Toku "Grace," "virtue," "reward," the blessings of heaven and earth that can be accumulated by a simple way of eating and other balanced practice.

Tokugawa The Japanese era from 1614-1868 during which the country enjoyed tranquil isolation from the rest of the world.

Un mei "Moving fortune" or "carrying destiny," the present spiritual direction of our life.

Yin and yang The law of universal change; the forces and tendencies that differentiate from one infinity and manifest as centrifugal and centripetal energy, space and time, and are the origin of all relative worlds.

Zen "Meditation," a form of Buddhism, especially popular in Japan, that emphasizes sudden enlightenment and simplicity in daily life.

129

Further Reading

Fukuoka, Masanobu. *The Natural Way of Farming*. Tokyo & New York: Japan Publications, Inc., 1985.

----------. *The Road Back to Nature*. Tokyo & New York: Japan Publications, Inc., 1987.

---------- *The One-Straw Revolution*. Emmaus, Pa.: Rodale Press, 1978.

Jack, Gale and Alex. *Promenade Home: Macrobiotics and Women's Health*. Tokyo & New York: Japan Publications, Inc., 1988.

Kaibara, Ekiken. *Yojokun: Japanese Secrets of Good Health*. Tokyo: Tokuma Shoten, 1974.

Kushi, Aveline, with Alex Jack. *Aveline Kushi's Complete Guide to Macrobiotic Cooking*. New York: Warner Books, 1985.

---------. *Aveline: The Life and Dream of the Woman Behind Macrobiotics Today*. Tokyo & New York: Japan Publications, Inc., 1988.

Kushi, Michio, with Edward Esko, *Natural Healing Through Macrobiotics*. Tokyo & New York: Japan Publications, Inc., 1978.

----------. *Nine Star Ki,* Becket, Mass.: One Peaceful World Press, 1991.

Kushi, Michio, with Alex Jack. *The Book of Macrobiotics: The Universal Way of Health, Happiness, and Peace*. Tokyo & New York: Japan Publications, Inc., 1986 (Revised Edition).

----------. *The Cancer-Prevention Diet*. New York: St. Martin's Press, 1983.

----------. *Diet for a Strong Heart*. New York: St. Martin's Press, 1985.

----------. *One Peaceful World*. New York: St. Martin's Press, 1987.

Kushi, Michio and Aveline, with Alex Jack. *Macrobiotic Diet*. Tokyo & New York: Japan Publications, Inc., 1985.

Macrobiotic Resources

For further information on macrobiotic classes and activities, including courses with Michio and Aveline Kushi and their associates please contact the Kushi Institute of the Berkshires in Becket, Massachusetts. Every month or every other month in Becket, Michio offers Spiritual Development Training Seminars and Study of Destiny Seminars incorporating Mizuno's principles on the way of eating, advanced teachings on physiognomy, and way of life practices associated with the *sennin*, or free human beings.

Kushi Institute
Box 7
Becket, Mass. 01223
(413) 623-5742

One Peaceful World is an international macrobiotic communications network and friendship society of individuals, families, centers, communities, businesses, and other organizations devoted to creating a healthy, peaceful world. One Peaceful World sponsors tours to East and West, forums and assemblies, and publishes a newsletter, books, videos, and other study materials. For membership information, contact:

One Peaceful World
Box 10
Becket, Mass. 01223
(413) 623-5742

About the Editors

Michio Kushi, the leader of the international macrobiotic community was born in Japan and studied international law and political science at Tokyo University. He came to the United States in 1949 and is the founder and chairman of the Kushi Institute, the Kushi Foundation, and One Peaceful World. He has given seminars on Oriental medicine and philosophy at the United Nations and served as advisor to governments in Europe, Africa, and Latin America. He is the author of several dozen books and lives with his wife in Becket and Brookline, Massachusetts.

Aveline Kushi came to the United States in 1951 after serving as an elementary school teacher in the mountains of central Japan. Erewhon, the pioneer natural foods company, began in her kitchen. Today she guides thousands of cooks each year through the many Kushi Institutes and macrobiotic centers and summer camps throughout the world. She is the mother of five children, grandmother of seven, and author of several books including her autobiography, *Aveline: The Dream of the Woman Behind Macrobiotics Today*.

Alex Jack has a background in writing and journalism, traveling to Vietnam, Russia, and China. For the last fifteen years, he has taught macrobiotics, serving as editor-in-chief of the *East West Journal,* director of the Kushi Institute of the Berkshires, and coordinator of One Peaceful World. His books include *Macrobiotic Diet* (with Michio and Aveline), *Promenade Home* (with Gale Jack), and *The New Age Dictionary*. He lives with his wife in Becket, Massachusetts.

Index